The Healthiest Meals on Earth

The Healthiest Meals on Earth

The Surprising, Unbiased Truth
About What Meals You Should Eat and Why

Jonny Bowden Ph.D., C.N.S., with Jeannette Bessinger

FAIR WINDS
PRESS
BEVERLY, MASSACHUSETTS

Text © 2008 Jonny Bowden

First published in the USA in 2008 by
Fair Winds Press, a member of
Quayside Publishing Group
100 Cummings Center
Suite 406-L
Beverly, MA 01915-6101
www.fairwindspress.com

12 11 10 09   9 10 11 12

ISBN-13: 978-1-59233-318-9
ISBN-10: 1-59233-318-4

Library of Congress Cataloging-in-Publication Data
Bowden, Jonny.
    The healthiest meals on earth : the surprising, unbiased truth about what meals you should eat and why / Jonny Bowden with Jeannette Bessinger.
        p. cm.
    Includes index.
    ISBN 1-59233-318-4
    1. Cookery (natural foods) 2. Low-carbohydrate diet — Recipes. I. Bessinger, Jeannette. II. Title.
    TX741.B635 2008
    641.5'636—dc22

Cover design: Dutton & Sherman
Book design: Kathie Alexander
Photography: Glenn Scott Photography, except where noted. iStockphoto: 2, 29, 30, 32–33, 48, 52–53, 76, 78–79, 93, 94, 98, 100–101, 111, 117, 122–123, 136, 140–141, 156, 160–161, 176, 180–181, 195, 200–201, 217, 222–223, 247, 248, 254–255, 271, 273, 278–279, 306, 312–313, 333, 336–337, 352, 357
Food Stylist: Catrine Kelty
Printed and bound in Singapore

The information in this book is for educational purposes only. It is not intended to replace the advice of a physician or medical practitioner. Please see your health-care provider before beginning any new health program.

To my mother, *Vivienne Simon Bowden*,

who taught me everything I know about cooking,

and to my partner and friend, *Jeannette Bessinger*,

who filled in the gaps

CONTENTS

INTRODUCTION /**8**

1 | Four-Course Polymeals /**22**

CHAPTER 1   **Fabulous Fiber:** Black Bean Cakes
with Cooling Accompaniments /**25**

CHAPTER 2   **Hunter-Gatherer's Delight:** Wild
Mushroom–Crusted Sirloin /**45**

CHAPTER 3   **Omega Star:** Broiled Salmon with
Tamari-Orange Marinade /**67**

CHAPTER 4   **Anti-Inflammatory Immune-System Booster:** Delicious
Dal with Sweet Onion and Curried Greens /**91**

CHAPTER 5   **Healthy Fats and Protein Packed:** Thai-Spiced Mango
and Prawns /**115**

CHAPTER 6   **Antioxidants from the Aegean:** Striped Bass with
Sun-Dried Tomato and Kalamata Paste /**135**

CHAPTER 7   **Iron Power:** Calf's Liver and Green Onions /**153**

CHAPTER 8   **Nourishing and Nutrient-Filled:** Persian-Style Chicken
with Walnut, Onion, and Pomegranate Sauce /**173**

CHAPTER 9   **Natural Protein Power:** Portobello
Buffalo Tenderloin /**193**

CHAPTER 10   **Healthiest Holiday Meal:** Citrus-Stuffed
Herbed Turkey /**213**

2 | One-Pot Polymeals with Simple Sides /242

CHAPTER 11   **The Healthiest Meat One-Pots Meals** /245

CHAPTER 12   **The Healthiest Poultry and Fish One-Pots Meals** /269

CHAPTER 13   **The Healthiest Vegetarian One-Pots Meals** /301

3 | Delicious Drinks: The Liquid Polymeal /324

CHAPTER 14   **The Healthiest Beverages** /327

RESOURCES /351

Food Chart of the Healthiest
Ingredients on Earth /351

The Right Oil for the Job /356

Sources for Specialty Ingredients /358

ACKNOWLEDGMENTS /359

INDEX /360

I want to start this introduction by telling you about something that you've probably never heard of before—the polymeal.

First, a bit of background. On June 28, 2003, a couple of research scientists (Nicholas Wald and Malcolm Law, if you really want to know) published a paper in the august *British Medical Journal* called "A Strategy to Reduce Cardiovascular Disease by More Than Eighty Percent." Because cardiovascular disease is the number-one killer in the United States, and most people would prefer to live longer and healthier, anything written by reputable scientists in a reputable medical journal that promises an 80 percent reduction in this deadly disease is going to get some serious attention.

Wald and Law theorized that if there was some way to combine a bunch of well-known, cheap medications into one hypothetical pill (which they called "the polypill"), and if you could somehow get everyone over 55 to take that pill every day, the reduced mortality from heart disease and stroke would be about 80 percent. This was only a statistical prediction, of course, but it was based on considerable research with large groups of people (like the famous Framingham Heart Study) that allowed them to predict how many people would normally die of cardiovascular disease over a given period of time, and how many would actually be saved by taking the polypill.

The polypill they proposed would contain a mix of six basic medications: three blood pressure medications plus a statin drug (which lowers cholesterol and inflammation), aspirin, and the B vitamin folic acid.

Which brings me to the polymeal.

FROM PILL TO PLATE

A year after the polypill was proposed, a Colombian scientist named Oscar Franco published a "reply" paper in the same *British Medical Journal*. Franco and his colleagues took the (gasp) revolutionary approach that maybe pills weren't the only way you could prevent disease. He suggested that dining regularly on a polymeal—a meal composed of ingredients that could boost the health of the heart and the blood vessels—could do just as good a job, cutting the risk of cardiovascular disease by more than three-quarters.

Using the same statistical prediction techniques as the previous researchers, Franco said that eating a diet rich in polymeals would delay the average onset of a heart attack by 9 years for men and 8 years for women, and that because cardiovascular disease is the number-one cause of mortality in industrialized nations, this delay would wind up increasing the average lifespan by between 4.8 and 6.6 years. Men could expect to live free from cardiovascular disease for at least 9 years more than they would without eating polymeals, and women could expect to be heart-disease-free for an additional 8.1 years.

"The point we are trying to make is that it is not only through pills that you can prevent disease," said Franco. "The polymeal is a natural alternative." Franco pointed out in interviews that by exercising, not smoking, and eating the prescribed food within a balanced diet, a future of "pills and medicalization" could be avoided.

"The polymeal promises to be an effective, non-pharmacological, safe, cheap, and tasty alternative to reduce cardiovascular morbidity and increase life expectancy in the general population," he concluded.

The major ingredients of the polymeal? Simple. Fish, garlic, almonds, fruits, vegetables, and dark chocolate, all polished off with a nice little glass of red wine.

Which got me thinking.

WHAT HIPPOCRATES KNEW THAT WE DON'T

Ever since Hippocrates—the father of modern medicine—uttered his famous saying "Let thy food be thy medicine and thy medicine be thy food," we've known that food has healing properties. I wrote about this at length in my book *The 150 Healthiest Foods on Earth*, discussing the remarkable and awesome ability of chemicals in food to serve as protectors of cells, defenders against cancer, and boosters of immunity.

Antioxidants, anti-inflammatories, flavonoids, polyphenols, and dozens of other classes of chemical compounds in foods help the liver get rid of toxins, protect DNA from damage, keep the brain and heart healthy, improve mood, and improve circulation, keeping blood and oxygen freely flowing to brain, heart, and other tissues.

Protein in our food provides the building blocks out of which the body constructs muscles, bones, neurotransmitters, and hormones; plant foods provide antioxidants and anti-inflammatories; and fats provide energy as well as anti-inflammatory and immune-enhancing properties of their own. No wonder people (like me) think of the local farmers' market as the ultimate natural pharmacy!

Homemade Energy Bars Yield: 12 bars
Your polymeal on the go

The energy bar recipe below is a perfect example of a portable polymeal—it's packed with protein, good fats in the form of nuts, and nutrient-rich apricots and raisins. If you're looking for an easy, nutritionally dense snack that travels well, this fits the bill perfectly.

Developed by pro triathlete Christy Underdonk, Potomac, Maryland

¼ cup (40 g) almonds

1½ cups (120 g) rolled oats (not instant)

1 cup (100 g) puffed brown rice cereal

1½ cups (263 g) diced dried apricots

1½ cups (220 g) currants or raisins

½ cup (64 g) nonfat vanilla protein powder

½ cup (56 g) toasted wheat germ

1 cup (340 g) brown rice syrup

½ cup (170 g) blue agave nectar

½ cup (130 g) reduced-fat peanut butter

1½ teaspoons vanilla extract

½ teaspoon cinnamon

Preheat oven to 350°F (180°C, gas mark 4).

Chop up the almonds by hand or put in a food processor and pulse a few times. Spread the oats, cereal, and almonds on a 13-× 9-inch (33- × 23-cm) nonstick pan lined with parchment paper. Bake, stirring occasionally, until the oats are toasted, about 15 minutes.

Meanwhile, chop the apricots, using a food processor if possible; transfer to a large bowl. Add the currants, protein powder, and wheat germ; toss with a rubber spatula to mix.

Combine the rice syrup and agave nectar in a heavy saucepan over medium-high heat and bring to a boil. Reduce the heat to low and stir in the peanut butter, vanilla, and cinnamon. Quickly pour the syrup over the oatmeal mixture and stir well.

With a spatula, immediately spread the warm mixture into a jelly-roll pan. Place another piece of parchment paper on top of the mixture and press into a thin, even layer. You must work quickly to prevent the mixture from becoming too cool and difficult to spread. Chill until firm, at least 4 hours.

Cut into 2- × 3-inch (5- × 8-cm) bars or whatever size desired. Wrap individually in plastic or foil and store in an airtight container and refrigerate. They can also be frozen for longer storage.

The Low-Fat Diet Myth

If you glance through the book, you may notice the presence of a number of ingredients such as coconut oil, avocado, and butter, which may surprise you. You—like most people—may have been taught to believe that such foods don't belong in a "healthy foods" book because they are high in fat.

Let me explain.

I do not believe in low-fat diets. I also do not believe that fat is at the root of all evil.

I realize this puts me in the outlier class of nutritionists, though there are more and more of us—doctors, nutritionists, naturopaths, and science journalists—who are coming on board every day. And I also realize that we may not become the "majority" opinion for many years. But hear me out anyway.

If you look deeply at the evidence—and I mean deeply, not as in "what's on the news?" but as in "what do the studies really show?"—you'll see that the evidence for low-fat diets preventing disease (even obesity) is pretty thin. You'll also see that the percentage of fat in the diet isn't related to any major health outcome, something that was pointed out by arguably the most prestigious nutritional epidemiologist of our time, Walter Willett, M.D., chairman of the nutrition department at the Harvard School of Public Health and lead researcher on the Nurses' Health Study, which essentially followed about 80,000 women over 30 years. No, fat doesn't cause disease.

But, in my humble opinion, sugar does.

The Fat versus Sugar Debate

Yup, I'm one of those crusty curmudgeons who thinks that when we bought the "fat is Satan" theory we were essentially buying VHS over BetaMax. The theory with the better public relations effort won, but it wasn't the better theory.

Sugar raises insulin, processed carbs raise insulin, high-fructose corn syrup raises insulin, and an unhealthy elevated level of insulin is turning out to be a major player not only in diabetes and obesity but in cancer, heart disease, erectile dysfunction, and Alzheimer's. The Atkins Diet may not have provided the perfect solution, but it was on to something—it's next to impossible to have good health and freedom from degenerative diseases without controlling blood sugar (and the insulin levels that high blood sugar creates).

Now this is not the place to get into this. (If you want the fullest, most conscientious account of how we came to mistake fat for the enemy while giving sugar a pass, read the most important nutrition book of the past ten years, *Good Calories, Bad Calories*, by my friend Gary Taubes.)

The point is this: We did not try to reduce fat in this book. Sure, there are a couple of low-fat options because I realize fat remains a big concern for many, many people, but I want you to know that the reason butter, coconut oil, eggs, avocados, and other healthy fats exist in this book is because there is nothing inherently unhealthy about them. What you will not see—or will see only the slightest, minimal use of—is sugar.

There, that's my prejudice. Call me crazy, but if you (and I) are around fifty years from now, I think you'll be calling me "right."

PERFECT MEAL

I began thinking about constructing meals as close as possible to the theoretically "perfect" meal that Franco talked about in the *British Medical Journal*. Since even the most dedicated person would eventually get tired of the same meal with the same seven ingredients (although that's hard to imagine when you're talking about chocolate), the meals would have to have as much variety as possible while being true to the "principles" of the polymeal. The ideal meal would maximize intake of anti-inflammatories, antioxidants, fiber, good fat, protein, vitamins, minerals, and plant chemicals (like resveratrol in grapes and wine or cacao in chocolate) that had been shown to improve some measure associated with health (like lowering blood pressure, for example, or reducing the risk of cancer).

In addition, since the best meal in the world isn't any good if no one eats it, the meals would have to be relatively easy (and fun) to make, and most of all delicious.

Which presented a bit of a problem, since I really don't cook very well. Okay, actually, I really don't cook *at all*.

So I turned to my lifelong friend, Jeannette Bessinger.

THAT'S WHAT FRIENDS ARE FOR

Let me tell you a little about Jeannette for three reasons. One, because she's just so interesting. Two, because she won't tell you most of this stuff herself. And three, because she's the one who developed the amazing recipes in this book, and I thought you'd enjoy them even more if you knew a bit about her.

I first met Jeannette when she was seventeen years old, and we have been friends for more years than I'm allowed to say because then you'd know her age and she'd have to kill me. When I met her, she had just graduated from a tough prep school in crusty Newport, Rhode Island, a school that she attended on full scholarship. Soon after, she was deciding on colleges—a hard decision, because Brown and Columbia had offered her full scholarships. (Brains were not in short supply in the Bessinger home.)

Long story short, after graduating from Columbia she went to an interfaith seminary where she became ordained as a nondenominational minister. She proceeded to spend the next ten years rigorously studying various healing paths, and that led her ultimately to the study of natural foods and nutrition.

For the last two decades, she has been putting her multiple talents to work doing things like starting and running award-winning theater programs for at-risk teens and counseling at-risk mothers and lower-income families on healthy eating and self-care. Spirituality and food have always figured big in her life. A part of that work has been with overweight women and their families. In venues ranging from hospitals to Head Start, she's taught a wide variety of people about food, health, shopping for ingredients, recipes, and meal preparation. Along the way she cowrote an amazing cookbook called *Whole Life Nutrition: A Simple Approach to Nourishing America's Busy Families,* which focuses on fresh, whole foods, healthy ingredients, delicious recipes, and most of all, ease of preparation.

Working with busy people who don't have the luxury (or the inclination) to spend all day in the kitchen preparing food yet who care deeply about making the best nutritional decisions for their families made Jeannette quite the expert on the care and feeding of families. She's now much in demand as a consultant and real foods chef, and I probably won't be able to afford her services after this book.

So I turned to Jeannette to work with me on the nuts-and-bolts portion of this book. We had wonderful assistance and original recipe contributions from such valued members of my team as Regina Wilshire and Lora Ruffner (not to mention the always invaluable input and help from my cherished assistants, clinical nutritionists Susan Mudd, M.S., C.N.S., and Suzanne Copp, M.S.). Regina is a naturopath with an encyclopedic knowledge of food and nutrition, and Lora is an experienced cook who owns the website www.lowcarbluxury.com and is well-versed in low-sugar cooking. Jeannette created, developed, wrote, or tweaked the vast majority of the recipes in this book.

And let me tell you, they are amazing.

A POLYMEAL COOKBOOK

I explained to Jeannette the concept of the polymeal and what I was after in putting the ideal meals together. We both agreed that each meal should feature a mix of ingredients that were selected on three criteria: one, maximizing nutritional impact; two, taste; and three, relative ease of preparation. By maximizing nutritional impact I mean using foods that are off the charts in terms of their ability to affect health by providing anti-inflammatories and antioxidants, vitamins and minerals, phytochemicals, fiber, protein, and healthy fat—like the energy bar recipe I've included in this introduction.

Although every single meal doesn't contain the seven magic ingredients of the original polymeal—red wine, chocolate, almonds, garlic, fish, fruits, and vegetables—our intention was to include ingredients in every meal that mimicked the effects of those seven touchstone ingredients and duplicated their health effects.

I think we succeeded. I hope you do, too.

Notes from the Chef

As a minister, nutrition educator, and lifestyle coach, I've worked with people of all ages from all walks of life who struggle with challenges to their health and wellness that many of us will face at one time or another.

I designed and currently facilitate a hospital-based lifestyle change program. One of the most successful aspects of the program (for improving health outcomes) is our approach to food and diet. We support people to leave the junk behind and start cooking and eating high-quality, nutrient-dense foods as a daily habit.

When Jonny Bowden and I were discussing the components of the healthiest meals on earth, we both agreed that all the ingredients should be of the highest quality. So we encourage you whenever possible to choose fresh, whole, organic plant foods and meats, eggs, and cheese from animals that have been treated humanely and raised organically on pasture.

Customize Your Cuisine

The healthiest meals are also quite bioindividual, meaning that what's the best meal for you today may not ultimately be the best meal for me. Or even the best meal for you tomorrow, because our nutritional needs change in subtle and not-so-subtle ways all the time. So it was important to offer a lot of variety in the menus in this book.

You can think of these meals and recipes as templates more than set formulas: Feel free to customize them so they fit your particular needs and palate. With the exception of baking (where dropping one little ingredient can make the whole thing die a horrible death), whole foods cooking is generally very forgiving and lends itself to experimentation.

The meals have actually been designed so that the sides, salads, and dessert dishes are somewhat interchangeable. We even provide you with "Suggested Swaps," which offer two good alternatives for that particular dish from the recipe collection.

What Is and Isn't on the Menu

In keeping with the polymeal concept, the healthiest meal "formula" should make good sense to you: Each of the meals contains some form of protein, fiber, healthy fat, and several foods that hit nutrient home runs. You will also see nuts or nut oils included or suggested in each meal.

What you will not see is any of the killer "whites": white rice, white flour, white sugar, or even white potatoes. We avoid them like the plague because nutritionally and metabolically, they all add up to the same thing: They disrupt blood sugar levels by raising insulin, which, as Jonny says in the intro, is probably the root cause of many of our growing national health problems. There is less than 1 cup (110 g) of (whole grain!) flour in all the recipes combined, and only ½ teaspoon of sucanat (a less processed form of sugar).

When writing the first book, Jonny reached out to his diverse and talented group of colleagues for their favorite recipes for the healthiest foods, so I started with some of those. I also called on my own team for a few of their inspirations. The rest are my original creations with your best health in mind. This smorgasbord provides you with a diverse, eclectic recipe collection designed to both inspire you and expand your daily repertoire.

There's something in here for everyone. If you happen to be a wild-game hunter, I hope you'll try a vegetarian dish. If you're a vegan, I hope you'll try a raw recipe. We've attempted to highlight as many different fabulous foods as possible and showcase a variety of preparation techniques, some of which may be new to you, like making raw soups or steam baking with the Schlemmertopf.

(continued on p. 20)

(continued from p. 19)

Section by Section

There are ten four-course meals, which necessarily require a little more preparation and provide you with a spectacular spread, including a selection of unique and healthy desserts (because we both firmly believe that food should be at least partly about pure pleasure). In chapter 10, we offer you a special holiday meal that is rich in both great flavors and awesome nutrition.

Beginning in chapter 11, there are ten one-pot polymeals with suggested simple sides for lighter fare or those busier times when you just want to get in and out of the kitchen more quickly. They are consistent with the polymeal "formula," providing you with all the nutrient-dense components of the four-course meals, just in a more compact form.

We close the book with a wonderful chapter about drinks, because the liquids we take in are as important as the foods we eat. Jonny highlights some of the most nourishing drinks out there, including red wine, special fruit juices, and "green" drinks. We even give you a formula for a power-packed smoothie: the liquid polymeal.

You will find a few preparation tips in the meal's introduction, and each recipe is followed by "Notes from the Kitchen." These are hints, tips, and tricks to help you work with these delicious foods on a regular basis. All the chapters are scored throughout with loads of sidebars on useful topics such as grass-fed beef, five great ways to prepare tofu, and the best oils for the best purposes to give you even more to chew on.

We hope you will enjoy these meals as much as we have enjoyed designing them for you.

Yours in gratitude,
Jeannette Bessinger

IT'S ALL ABOUT YOU

If there's one sensibility that informs every single book and article I've written, every workshop or lecture I've given, every radio show I've hosted, it's this: It's all about the person. As Lance Armstrong says, "It's not about the bike." It's not about the diet, it's about the *dieter*. Health is not about the illness, it's about the *patient*. Wealth is not about the investments, it's about the *investor*.

As I've said many times, Western medicine asks the question "What is this illness?" but Eastern (holistic) medicine asks a different question: "Who is this person before me?"

So while this book is about food and food preparation, I want you to know that it's really about you the *preparer*. There's a big school of thought that says that part of the many reasons food can be so healing is because of love. It's hard not to put love and care and consciousness into the preparation of "slow food" (meaning stuff you don't actually buy and eat in a drive-through). And consciousness is the best friend of a person trying to be healthy, as it is the best friend of a person trying to do just about anything well.

I hope this book gives you useful, valuable, and wonderful information, but I also hope it helps you become more conscious and involved with your food. After all, it is truly your best medicine. With it, you can heal almost anything, or—at the very least—make something in your life better.

Enjoy the journey!

Jonny Bowden
Los Angeles, October 2007

1 | Four-Course Polymeals

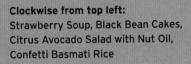

Clockwise from top left:
Strawberry Soup, Black Bean Cakes,
Citrus Avocado Salad with Nut Oil,
Confetti Basmati Rice

Fabulous Fiber

Black Bean Cakes with Cooling Accompaniments

MEAL:

34 Black Bean Cakes

36 Confetti Basmati Rice

38 Citrus Avocado Salad
   with Nut Oil

40 Strawberry Soup

THIS MEAL is a vegetarian delight that even a meat lover could love. The grains/beans/seeds combo provides quality vegetarian protein, meaning it contains all of the essential amino acids (always a challenge for vegetarians). The meal is low glycemic (more on that in a moment), loaded with healthy fats, and high in fiber. And the dessert is as delicious as it sounds. What could be bad?

BEANS FOR BLOOD SUGAR BALANCE

The centerpiece of the entrée is black beans in the delicious Black Bean Cakes. I've written extensively—in *The 150 Healthiest Foods on Earth* and countless articles—about the importance of keeping blood sugar smack in the middle of what my friend Barry Sears, M.D., calls "The Zone." Remember Goldilocks tasting her porridge? ("Not too hot, not too cold … just right.") Well that's how you want your blood sugar. If you drew a picture of how your blood sugar fluctuates during the day, you'd want it to look like a nice rolling lake in the summer, not like a tidal wave in the Pacific. Most people eating the standard American diet would have a blood sugar "graph" that looked like the latter, not the former.

I'm fond of saying that when you eat a bagel (or any food that contains a lot of sugar or converts to sugar quickly) your blood sugar skyrockets to the ceiling (think "tidal wave"). Beans are the ultimate "low glycemic" food, meaning their effect on your blood sugar is slow, gradual, and gentle (think "rolling lake").

Why is this important? Because high levels of blood sugar produce high levels of *insulin*, the fat-storing hormone. And because what goes up must come down, high levels of blood sugar also generally result in a big old crash, leaving you with cravings, hunger, and a ravenous desire for more carbohydrates, which will push your blood sugar back up, starting the whole cycle over again. Meanwhile, you rarely feel good, your energy and mood suffer, you're not a lot of fun to be around, and it's fiendishly difficult to lose weight.

Sound familiar?

Meal Prep Tips

- The beans and rice have extended cooking times, so begin with these items. Set both to soak in the morning or overnight and start the meal preparation with the beans.

- When beans are on the stove, prepare the rice.

- The salad and dessert can be assembled while the beans and rice are cooking, or you can prepare the dessert soup after you eat because the prep time is minimal.

THE NUMBER ONE WEIGHT-LOSS SUPPLEMENT

The reason beans are such a great low glycemic food can be summed up in one word: fiber. When I wrote *Living the Low Carb Life*, I included a chapter on weight-loss supplements in which I said that almost none of them did any good (I've since amended that—see *The Most Effective Natural Cures on Earth*). What I'd now say is that *very few* of them do any good. The exception is what I call the number one supplement for weight loss—fiber.

Fiber's not expensive, it's not sexy, and it's not exotic, but it works like a charm, and beans are one of the best sources on the planet. There are at least a dozen clinical studies that have linked fiber with weight loss. Fiber makes you feel full and therefore less likely to overeat. It suppresses hunger. It enhances blood-sugar control and insulin effects and—according to the *CRC Handbook of Dietary Fiber in Human Nutrition*, fiber can even reduce the number of calories that the body absorbs—translating into a 3- to 18-pounds of weight loss per year by some estimates! Fiber rocks! And beans have got it.

BEANS' CELL-PROTECTING BENEFITS

Besides fiber, there are other compounds in beans that protect your health. One phytochemical in beans—called dysgenic—seems to inhibit cancer cells. Other phytochemicals—such as saponins, protease inhibitors, and physic acid—seem to protect cells from the kind of genetic damage that can lead to cancer later on. Saponins, for example, seem to inhibit the reproduction of cancer cells and also slow the growth of tumors. While all this lab stuff is interesting, more important is the simple fact that folks who eat beans have a reduced rate of cancer. An analysis of questionnaires in the famous Nurses' Health Study all found that women who consumed higher intakes of beans (or lentils) had a striking 24 percent reduced risk of breast cancer, and all that seemed to be needed was a minimum of two servings per week. And according to the American Institute of Cancer Research, *men* who eat the most beans have a 38 percent lower risk of prostate cancer than men who eat the least. Worth thinking about.

A PRODUCE BONANZA

The **Citrus Avocado Salad with Nut Oil** salad is built around one of my favorite foods—avocado. The poor avocado suffered from an unde-served bad reputation for so many years while the country was in the grips of the mass dietary hysteria that produced the low-fat movement, but thankfully we're coming to our senses and recognizing the overwhelming benefit of certain kinds of fat in our diet.

One of those healthful fats is monounsaturated fat—and avocado is loaded with it. Monounsaturated fat like the kind found in avocados is a big part of one of the healthiest diets in the world—the Mediterranean diet. Virtually every study has shown that people eating a Mediterranean diet—with its emphasis on fish, fruits, vegetables, nuts, and monounsatu-rated fat—have lower rates of heart disease. People following a modified low carb diet high in monounsaturated fat lost more weight than people following the standard National Cholesterol Education Program diet, according to research published in 2004 in the *Archives of Internal Medicine*. I've been known to eat half an avocado right out of the shell, just for a mini-meal. Delicious? Yes. Fattening? No. At least if you eat it instead of an equal number of calories of junk food.

The **Confetti Basmati Rice** contains a colorful mixture of red and yellow peppers (an excellent source of vitamins C and A), green onion, and parsley (or cilantro), plus toasted pumpkin seeds. These delicious seeds pack a nutritional wallop. They are a rich source of minerals, especially magnesium, potassium, and phosphorus. Interestingly, the roasted kind has far more protein, at least according to the U.S. Food and Drug Administration's food database. Read more about the benefits of rice in Chapter 11.

A SWEET DESSERT

The **Strawberry Soup** dessert is outstanding, and since the overall glycemic load of the meal is low, it's not likely to do much damage to your blood sugar. Yogurt—featured in the soup—is loaded with probotics, the beneficial bacteria that help keep your gut healthy and your digestive processes running smoothly. And another soup ingredient, raw honey, unlike that imposter that comes in the cute little squeezy bear, is a real food. It hasn't been heated, so the enzymes are intact, and it tastes way better than the homogenized, pasteurized imitators.

Enjoy!

Beans and Your Social Life

Beans are really good for you, but they may not make you the most popular houseguest. In fact, they could easily put a major damper on your social life.

Let's face it, some people just stay away from beans because digesting them—at least without certain embarrassing side effects—is difficult. But here's the thing—your system may simply need time to adjust to them, especially if they are a relatively new food in your diet or you eat them infrequently. You can minimize the digestive issues by adding beans to your weekly diet slowly. Some experts feel that by increasing the amount of beans you eat gradually, your system will get better at both producing "bean-breaking" enzymes and digesting beans.

Also, presoak and cook beans thoroughly: they must be tender to the squeeze. Undercooked beans are particularly hard to digest. Chewing them slowly and thoroughly will also help. Drink plenty of water between meals.

And don't forget Beano. Just as Lactaid helps you break down the lactose milk sugar in milk that causes problems for many people, Beano helps break down two of the sugars most responsible for forming gas—stachyrose and raffinose. Beano is basically a great natural over-the-counter enzyme product that can really help reduce gas.

Black Bean Cakes
Fiber-rich comfort food

Prep Time: 10 minutes
Cook Time: Soak overnight, approximately 70 minutes cooking time and 60 minutes refrigeration time

Ingredients

2 cups (1 lb, or 500g) dried black beans, picked over and rinsed, soaked overnight and drained

½ teaspoon cumin

4 cups (940 ml) water or broth (one 32-oz carton, organic, no-sodium-added, vegetable or chicken broth)

8 medium cloves garlic, finely minced

½ cup (8 g) fresh cilantro, chopped

½ teaspoon salt

1 to 2 tablespoons (15-30 ml) extra virgin olive oil

1 cup (520 g) salsa, any variety, optional

Combine the black beans, cumin, and water or broth in a large saucepan over high heat. Bring to a boil. Reduce heat to low, partially cover, and simmer until beans are tender (60 to 70 minutes). Drain well.

In a large bowl, mash the beans and garlic together well. Stir in the cilantro and salt. Form the mixture into eight cakes. Transfer to a plate and refrigerate for one hour.

In a large, nonstick frying pan, heat the olive oil over medium heat. Add the cakes and cook, turning over once, until warmed and the outside is slightly crisp, about 5 to 7 minutes. Serve immediately with salsa on the side. Leftovers keep well for 2 to 3 days.

Yield: 8 servings

Notes from the Kitchen

- If you don't have time to cook beans from scratch, use 5 cups canned organic beans, rinsed and drained.

- To remove the lingering smell of garlic or onion from your hands, rinse with a stainless steel "soap" bar and water. A steel soap bar is a piece of stainless steel in the shape of a soap bar. Holding the bar under running water and rubbing your hands and fingertips along its surface helps to more efficiently remove the lingering odors of strong foods like garlic and onions. The shape itself isn't important—any piece of stainless steel will accomplish the same thing. You can purchase a steel soap at most kitchen goods supply stores for $5 to $10.

- A garlic press is a handy tool for quickly mincing lots of cloves. If you don't have one, try putting an unpeeled clove under a vegetable scraper and leaning down on it with the flat of your hand to crush it. The meat will come easily out the skin and you can mince further with a sharp knife, if necessary.

- Use non-Teflon, nonstick pans for reduced oil sautéing or healthy "frying."

Canned versus Dried Beans

- Cooking your own beans is cheaper than buying canned beans. Home-cooked beans taste fresher, plus no vitamins, minerals, or enzymes are destroyed by pre-cooking or canning.

- For busy individuals or families, canned beans are still a great option. But read the labels: choose beans that are organic and free of added salt, msg, or preservatives.

Confetti Basmati Rice

A vitamin and mineral packed side dish

Prep Time: 10 minutes
Cook Time: 1 hour

Ingredients

1 cup (195 g) brown basmati rice, well rinsed (and soaked, optional)

¼ cup (35 g) raw or toasted pumpkin seeds

2 cups (470 ml) water or broth (no-sodium-added vegetable or chicken broth)

Pinch salt

½ red pepper, diced into squares (see Notes from the Kitchen)

½ yellow or orange pepper, diced into squares (see Notes from the Kitchen)

¼ cup (4 g) flat leaf parsley or cilantro, washed and coarsely chopped

1 bunch green onion stalks, diced into ½ inch pieces, bulbs removed

Zest from half a lime or lemon

2 tablespoons (30 ml) fresh squeezed lime (about 1 lime) or lemon juice (about half a lemon)

Add the rice, seeds, water or broth, and salt to a medium saucepan with a tight-fitting lid. (You can also use same proportions in a rice cooker, set for brown rice.) Bring to a boil and stir once. Reduce the heat to low, cover, and simmer for about 50 minutes. Remove from heat without removing lid. Allow to sit covered for 10 minutes.

While the rice is resting, core and seed the peppers. Dice them into small, ½-inch squares. Clean and chop the cilantro and green onion stalks. Zest the lemon or lime, cut it, and squeeze the juice. Fold all ingredients gently into the rice until well-combined.

Serve immediately. Leftovers keep well for 2 to 3 days.

Yield: 8 servings (about 3 cups [675 g] in total)

Suggested Swaps

• Steam-Baked Vidalia Onions (page 104)
• Fragrant Chard (page 204)

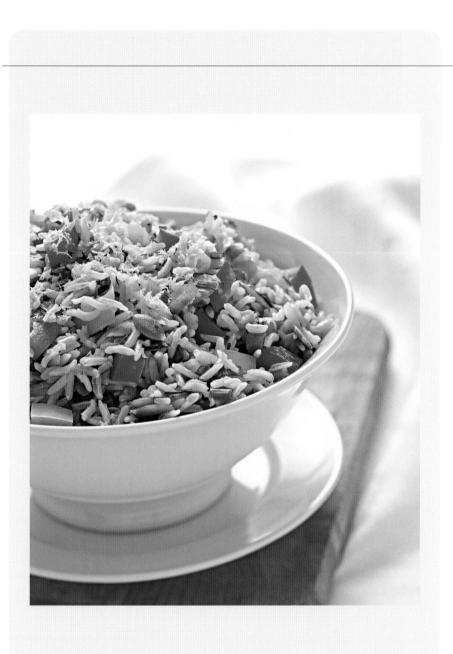

Notes from the Kitchen

- Basmati is an aromatic rice with a dry grain that tends to stay separate rather than clump together. You must rinse it gently but thoroughly until the rinse water does not cloud.

- Store grains in the fridge if you have room, or freeze for three days in the freezer to kill meal moth eggs and then store in cool, dark pantry.

- Cutting pepper "confetti": Choose square-shaped peppers. Cut off the tops and bottoms and cut down one side on a "corner edge" to open the peppers. Neatly pull out the core and seeds. Cut the peppers into four square, flat pieces. Cut into ½-inch strips, then dice strips into ½-inch squares, removing any remaining white stalk.

Citrus Avocado Salad with Nut Oil

Rich in good fat and vitamin C

Prep Time: 5 to 10 minutes
Cook Time: None

Ingredients

1 ripe avocado, sliced into eighths

1 orange (blood orange, if available), peeled, cut in half, segments pulled apart

1 head Boston or butter lettuce, washed, cored, and leaves separated

1 tablespoon (15 ml) macadamia nut oil

1 teaspoon agave nectar or
½ teaspoon raw honey

1 tablespoon (15 ml) fresh lime juice
(½ lime squeezed well)

Lay out whole lettuce leaves to cover the surface of a platter. Arrange avocado slices on top of leaves. Fill in with orange segments. Whisk oil, sweetener, and lime juice together well. Drizzle dressing over top of salad. Serve immediately.

Yield: 4 generous servings

Suggested Swaps

• Veggie Slaw with Flax Oil (page 166)

• Crunchy Coconut Fruit Salad (page 126)

Notes from the Kitchen

- Speed the ripening process by placing the avocado in a brown paper bag with a banana or an apple. You can also wrap it in a warm towel and put it in the sun. Fruit ripens best in a warm, dark place.

- If you want to make a smaller salad and save half of the avocado, leave the pit in remaining half—it will help slow the browning process.

- To cut an avocado cleanly, insert a sharp knife along the length of the fruit and turn the fruit to make a neat, lengthwise cut through the middle. Twist the two halves apart and lay them down. Insert the tip of your knife or a sharp fork into the pit (while on the counter, not in your hand!) and, grasping the meat gently, twist the pit out of the avocado.

Strawberry Soup

Fortified with probiotic-rich yogurt

Prep Time: 5 to 10 minutes
Cook Time: None

Ingredients

2 heaping cups (290 g) strawberries,
   washed and stemmed (1 pint of fresh
   is best, or 2 cups frozen, thawed)
1½ cups (355 ml) cold water
¼ cup (60 ml) dry red wine, such
   as Merlot
¼ cup (85 g) raw honey
½ cup (115 g) plain yogurt
¼ teaspoon ground cardamom
Sliced berries or mint leaves for garnish,
   optional

Fill a 2-cup liquid measuring cup to overflowing with the strawberries. Rinse the berries, drain, and pour into a blender. Measure the cold water and wine into a measuring cup and add four ice cubes to chill further.

Puree the berries. Add the honey and yogurt and blend lightly until well mixed. Pour the strawberry mixture into a bowl. Gently stir in the water/wine mixture, straining through and discarding ice cubes. Stir in cardamom.

Serve very cold, garnished with a few sliced berries or mint leaves.

Yield: 6 servings

Suggested Swaps

- Grilled Pineapple (page 148)
- Tropical Frosties (page 130)

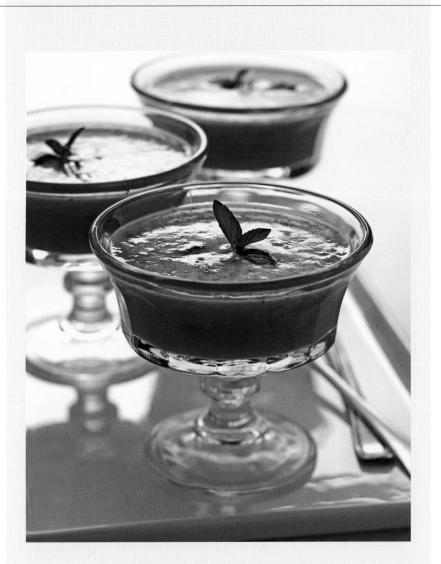

Notes from the Kitchen

- You can use other berries, such as blueberries or raspberries, for an equally delicious soup. Simply adjust the sweetener amounts to taste. A dry fruity white wine, such as a Chardonnay, Sauvignon Blanc, or a good Chablis, works well.

- Raw berry soups are the perfect finisher for pungent spicy dishes or hot summer nights.

Making Mexican Meals Healthier

Here are ways to increase the health benefits of Mexican food.

- Don't fry refried beans: boil and mash them instead, adding spices for flavor.

- Salsas are a great way to add fresh vegetables and fruits to a meal while sparking up its color and taste. So don't be afraid to experiment with different types.

- Avoid the starchy Spanish rice and choose a brown rice, or better yet, double up on the vegetables.

The "Dirty" Dozen of Food

The Environmental Working Group, a nonprofit research organization based in Washington, D.C., analyzed the results of nearly 43,000 Department of Agriculture and Food and Drug Administration tests for pesticides on produce conducted between 2000 and 2004.

The group found that the peaches and apples topped the list of most contaminated, with almost 97 percent of peaches testing positive for pesticides and almost 87 percent having two or more pesticide residues. Approximately 92 percent of apples tested positive, with 72 percent having two or more residues.

The following twelve fruits and vegetables were the most contaminated, the group found:

1. Peaches
2. Apples
3. Sweet bell peppers
4. Celery
5. Nectarines
6. Strawberries
7. Cherries
8. Pears
9. Imported grapes
10. Spinach
11. Lettuce
12. Potatoes

For these twelve foods, as well as with coffee, milk, poultry, and other meat, we recommend that you buy organic.

The counterpart to the Environmental Working Group's "Dirty Dozen" is their list of the twelve foods that are most consistently clean. Here they are:

1. Onions
2. Avocados
3. Sweet corn
4. Pineapples
5. Mango
6. Asparagus
7. Sweet peas
8. Kiwi
9. Bananas
10. Cabbage
11. Broccoli
12. Papaya

Of the three top foods on the "consistently clean" list—onions, avocados, and sweet corn—more than 90 percent of samples tested had no detectable pesticide residues!

Chapter 1 **Pantry List**

FOOD GROUP	FOOD
Dairy	Plain yogurt
Grains	Brown basmati rice
Herbs/Spices/Condiments	Cardamom (ground) Cilantro (fresh) Cumin Garlic Mint leaves (optional) Parsley (fresh) Salsa Salt
Miscellaneous	Agave nectar (or raw honey) Black beans (dried or canned) Olive oil (extra virgin) Raw honey Red wine (dry)
Nuts/Seeds	Macadamia nut oil Pumpkin seeds
Produce	Avocado Boston or butter lettuce Green onion stalks Limes or lemons Orange Orange or yellow pepper Strawberries (fresh or frozen)

Clockwise from top left:
Wild Mushroom–Crusted Sirloin,
Real-Food Brownies, Broccoli Rabe
with Raspberry-Vinegar Reduction,
Baby Spinach Salad with Fresh
Raspberries

CHAPTER 2

Hunter-Gatherer's Delight

Wild Mushroom-Crusted Sirloin

MEAL:

54 Wild Mushroom-
Crusted Sirloin

58 Baby Spinach Salad
with Fresh Raspberries

60 Broccoli Rabe with
Raspberry-Vinegar
Reduction

62 Real-Food Brownies

SOME PEOPLE might think, "What in the world is sirloin steak doing in a book on the healthiest meals on Earth?" So let's get the whole meat thing out of the way first.

IN DEFENSE OF MEAT

A ton of studies have linked animal products with increased risk for a number of diseases you don't want to have. Troubling studies link meat consumption with a number of cancers, and also with a greater incidence of Alzheimer's. But before you completely rule meat out of your diet, you should know that there are also problems with those studies, and certain details worth thinking about.

Most studies linking eating habits with diseases are investigating patterns of eating. A study in the August 15, 2007, issue of the *Journal of the American Medical Association* was reported in the media as finding that "diets high in fat and meat were linked to a higher risk for colon cancer," but when you read the study you found that it was the Western diet *as a whole* that was linked to higher rates of cancer, particularly when compared to a diet high in vegetables, nuts, and fiber. Sure, the Western diet is filled with meat, but it's generally of the ballpark frank kind rather than the pasture-fed organic kind. Not only that, but the Western diet is also very low in fiber, very high in sugar, very high in refined food in general, and very low in vegetables. And the fat tends to be of the kind found in French fries. Taken as a whole, that's a pretty dismal, disease-producing picture, but whether meat per se is to blame is another story.

I've always been of two minds about meat. I'm deeply concerned about animals and about the conditions under which they live and die on huge factory farms, which supply most of the meat you eat. The animals are fed grain, which is the wrong diet for cows that normally graze on pasture and grass. They're given tons of antibiotics, and they're fattened up with steroids and hormones, all of which get into their meat (and milk) and all of which you consume when you eat it. To top it off, most processed meats are loaded with carcinogenic nitrates, and many meats are grilled and charred, increasing their content of cancer-causing compounds. (See "To Grill or Not to Grill" on page 56.) Given the quality of most of the meat the average person eats, it's pretty darn hard to recommend it.

But the other side is that like it or not, most humans do better with some animal products in their diet. They just do. (Not everyone, granted, but most.) Meat is a great source of the most absorbable kind of iron, not to mention it's loaded with B vitamins. If you buy grass-fed, organic meat (see "Top Seven Reasons to Buy Grass-Fed Meat" in this chapter) you by-pass a lot of the problems that have been associated with meat eating. No antibiotics. No steroids. No nitrates. No hormones. And even better, when cows eat their natural diet of grass and pasture, their fat content is entirely different. Their omega-3 content is high, and their fat also contains cancer-fighting conjugated linolenic acid, a kind of fat that's virtually absent in the meat and fat of factory-farmed animals.

So that's why sirloin made it into this book, in this meal's main dish **Wild Mushroom–Crusted Sirloin**. If you're going to eat meat—and many people are—I suggest spending the extra money and getting the grass-fed kind. Just eat it less often. And surround it with vegetables, healthy fats, and all the other things that support your health.

Like the stuff that's in this meal.

A GIANT AMONG GREENS

Like spinach. Pound for pound, spinach—like many green leafy vegetables—provides more nutrients than almost any other food on the planet. (The possible exception might be sea algae, but no one eats that much of that.)

Spinach, superb in our **Baby Spinach Salad with Fresh Raspberries**, is a great source of an underappreciated vitamin that's essential for strong bones but that no one talks about much: vitamin K. Vitamin K actually activates a compound in your body called osteocalcin, whose job it is to anchor calcium molecules inside the bone. A cup of spinach contains 200 percent of the (too low!) Daily Value for vitamin K. Enjoy this salad and your bones will thank you!

Spinach, especially the way it's prepared in this meal, is downright delicious. (If you think I'm smoking something, wait until you try it.) Jeannette has put together a particular combination of flavors that not only is packed with nutrition, but that balances sweet and sour and crunchy and soft in a way that makes this salad taste almost like a dessert (okay, almost, but even so!). The nuts add healthy fat, the soft goat or feta cheese adds calcium and more protein, and the raspberries add sweetness and fiber, not to mention ellagic acid, which has been shown in animal research and laboratory models to inhibit the growth of certain kinds of tumors. And that's on top of raspberries' nice little helping of potassium, calcium, magnesium, vitamin C, and our old friend vitamin K. And the dressing is naturally sweet because of the juice-sweetened raspberry jam and the raw honey or agave nectar.

Broccoli rabe, the main event in **Broccoli Rabe with Raspberry-Vinegar Reduction**, is a bit of an acquired taste, but it's worth it. It's slightly bitter, but the raspberry vinegar balances it out nicely.

Broccoli rabe, which isn't really related to broccoli except in name, is more kin

Top Seven Reasons to Buy Grass-Fed Meat

1. No antibiotics added. Antibiotics are routinely given to cattle in factory farms to help manage the problems brought on by their highly concentrated grain diets and living conditions.

2. No steroids or growth hormones. Steroids or bovine growth hormones are routinely given to commercial beef to speed up growth and weight gain for faster "finishing" times. These hormones actually make it into your body and have been implicated in a number of health problems, including acne.

3. Contains healthy omega-3 fats. When cattle are fed their normal diet of pasture, their fat is different from that of their grain-fed, factory-farmed brethren—and it contains way more healthy omega-3 fats.

4. Contains conjugated linolenic acid (CLA). This healthy, cancer-fighting fat is made normally in the chambers of the bovine stomach. Grass-fed animals are a great source of CLA—grain-fed factory-farmed animals have next to none due to the high acidity of their stomachs.

5. Animals tended as humanely as possible to minimize stress and trauma. Organic farms—like U.S. Wellness Meats, for example—care deeply about their animals' quality of life.

6. Animals are fed no contaminated animal by-product feed. Serious, organic farmers raising cows on pasture simply don't feed their cattle animal by-products, reducing or eliminating the risk of contamination and conditions such as mad cow disease.

7. Minimal risk of *E. coli*. Grain-fed animals have a much higher level of acidity in their stomachs, which *E. coli* need to survive. Pasture-fed animals do not have an internal environment that's hospitable to *E. coli*.

Meal Prep Tips

- The Real-Food Brownies can be prepared ahead.

- The rub keeps for a very long time, so you can make it any time you have dried mushrooms on hand and store it in a tightly lidded container—a small glass jar with a screw top works great. No need to refrigerate; just keep it on the pantry shelf.

- The sirloin steaks should come out of the refrigerator first so they have about 30 minutes to rest at room temperature before grilling.

- Prepare the raspberry dressing and assemble the salad ingredients while the steaks are resting.

- Wash the broccoli rabe, prepare the steaks, and put the rabe and steaks on at about the same time.

- Dress the salad right before sitting down to eat.

to the turnip. It's a member of the Brassica family of vegetable royalty, which includes such heavyweights as cabbage and Brussels sprouts, and it contains plant compounds like sulforaphane, flavonoids, and indoles. Flavonoids are anti-inflammatory agents, and sulforaphane helps activate enzymes involved in detoxification. Indoles collectively help protect against cancer and also may help protect against the carcinogenic effect of pesticides and other toxins. What a trio!

THE MAGIC OF COCOA

If you look ahead and read the dessert recipe, **Real-Food Brownies**, you might do a double-take at first. Brownies made with garbanzo beans? Yup. And wait till you taste them. Not for nothing did we call them "real-food brownies." There's not a drop of white flour in them, and you might have noticed they're made without sugar.

What they do have is cocoa, which is emerging as one of the surprising health foods of the twenty-first century. Studies show that cocoa contains a particular subclass of flavonoids called flavanols, which prevent fatlike substances in the bloodstream from clogging up your arteries. That reduces the blood's ability to clot, which in turn reduces the risk of stroke and heart attack. And in what WebMD called "the best medical news in ages," studies in two important scientific journals—*Nature* and the *Journal of the American Medical Association*—show that the cocoa (or dark chocolate, which contains cocoa) can modestly lower blood pressure.

The flavanols in cocoa also turn up the body's production of an important compound called nitric oxide, which is so important for cardiovascular health, healthy blood pressure—and yes, guys—erections! (Viagra works by helping to turn on the nitric oxide faucet!)

And as for those garbanzo beans? You'll never know they're in there. Meanwhile, they create a high-fiber, heart-healthy dessert that will put a smile on your face.

Enjoy!

Cacao versus Cocoa: What's the Difference?

The terms cacao and cocoa are sometimes used interchangeably—there are no hard and fast rules. Technically, cacao refers to the raw, unprocessed pods that come from the actual cacao tree (*Theobroma cacao*), while cocoa refers to the product made when you shell the pods and ferment, dry, and roast the seeds. (The seeds don't start to smell chocolatey until they're fermented.)

With still more processing and the addition of ingredients like sugar, the cocoa turns into actual chocolate. Dark chocolate with the highest cocoa (or cacao) content—typically 70 percent—is the best kind.

The more cocoa (or cacao) it contains, the more health-giving plant compounds (like flavanols) it contains. Note: Actual pure cocoa is bitter. Chocolate with high cocoa content (80 percent and above) will be loaded with the healthy stuff but won't taste nearly as sweet as your typical candy bar.

Wild Mushroom–Crusted Sirloin

An all-natural, organic delicacy that fights cancer too

Prep Time: 15 minutes
Cook Time: 20 minutes

Ingredients

4 small sirloin steaks (5 to 6 ounces
   or 140 to 168 g each) or two
   12-ounce (340-g) steaks (1¼ pounds
   or 570 g total), pounded to less than
   1 inch (3 cm) thick and cut in half
½ ounce (15 g) dried wild or shiitake
   mushrooms
2 teaspoons red or black peppercorns
1½ teaspoons sea salt
½ teaspoon rapadura or other
   raw sugar
1 teaspoon high-heat vegetable oil,
   such as avocado
1 teaspoon extra virgin olive oil
1 bunch green onions, separated:
   ¼ cup (25 g) white section thinly
   sliced and ¼ cup (25 g) green section
   finely chopped
1 cup (235 ml) high-quality dry
   red wine

Gently rinse the steaks in water and pat dry.

In a coffee grinder, grind the mushrooms to powder and remove them to a bowl. Place the peppercorns, salt, and sugar in the grinder and grind them until a fine powder is achieved. Combine the 2 powders and mix well to make the rub "crust."

Lay the steaks out on a platter and brush them lightly on both sides with avocado oil. Gently pour ½ tablespoon of the powder onto the tops of each steak. Rub it lightly with your fingertips until the surface area is evenly covered. Flip the steaks and coat the other sides in the same manner.

Heat a heavy skillet with raised ridges over medium-high heat for about 4 minutes. Add the steaks to the skillet and sear for 3 to 4 minutes on each side, or until they are just springy to the touch for rare meat. Gently transfer the steaks with a slotted spatula to a platter and loosely cover them with a saucepan lid so they can continue to cook. Pour off any fat in the skillet.

Add the 1 teaspoon olive oil and white onion slices to the skillet, and sauté over medium heat, stirring, until softened.

Deglaze the skillet with the wine by gently pouring the wine into the pan, scraping up any remaining crust or other "bits," and bringing the mixture to a boil. Scrape the pan until it is smooth, and then stir the mixture occasionally as it cooks. Simmer the wine mixture until it is reduced to a thicker sauce or "glaze," usually 5 to 10 minutes. Remove the skillet from the heat and gently stir in the green scallions and salt and pepper to taste, if desired.

Spoon a bit of the wine sauce onto each of the 4 plates, cover with the steaks, and pour the remaining sauce over the tops.

Yield: 4 servings

Notes from the Kitchen

- You can also grill these steaks outdoors. A hot outdoor grill is superior to the oven broiler for sealing the crust and the juices inside. But be sure to read "To Grill or Not to Grill" on page 56 first!

- For the mushrooms, try porcini or morel for a stronger flavor, or maitake or shiitake for a more subtle flavor.

- A "high-heat" oil is cooking oil with a high smoking point; i.e., the temperature at which oil begins to smoke and break down. See "The Right Oil for the Job" on page 356 for more information about which oils are safest at which temperatures. Other possible choices are grapeseed or canola oil.

- Keep a small designated coffee grinder for powdering spices and other flavoring foods for rubs, dressings, and marinades. Oil from the coffee beans permeates delicate spices, so you can't use one machine for both purposes. Grinders are not expensive or large, so it's perfectly practical to own two.

- Buying spices whole prolongs their shelf life, and the flavor potency of a freshly ground spice is superior to the prepowdered form.

- Dried wild mushrooms can be pricey. But don't let that put you off. A little goes a long way. Try grinding them and using a small amount; you'll be surprised at how little it takes to infuse foods with wonderful earthy flavors. Chef Sally Schneider (*A New Way to Cook*) suggests powdering the mushrooms and adding salt, pepper, and a pinch of sugar to make a dry rub.

- Store the remaining powder in a tightly sealed jar for a later use. The rub will keep as long as the shelf life of the mushrooms you used, up to a couple of months.

- The caps of mushrooms contain more nutrients than the stems.

To Grill or Not to Grill

Grilling is as American as apple pie, but like a lot of things we've always assumed were healthy, it's come under fire recently for presenting some serious health risks.

Grilling raises two concerns, both of them because of chemical reactions. One of these happens when fat drips on the coals and forms nasty little compounds called polycyclic aromatic hydrocarbons or PAHs, which are carcinogenic. Good as that black stuff tastes on the charred meats and fish, it's loaded with PAHs. Avoid flaming, charring, or blackening, and should it happen, just scrape off the black stuff.

The other—and possibly bigger—problem is a chemical reaction that happens inside of animal foods (meat, chicken, or other poultry) that are kept on the grill for a long time at high temperatures. Compounds inside the food react to high temperatures and create heterocyclic amines (HCAs), which have been shown to trigger tumors in mice. More than two dozen studies have shown a troubling link between cancer and high consumption of these well-done, grilled foods.

Open flames are needed to make PAHs, but any high-temperature heat source—propane, for example—can form HCAs. You can reduce the formation of PAHs by not exposing food directly to the heat source and the resulting smoke while grilling. And you can reduce the formation of HCAs by not leaving meat on the grill (or flame) for a long time. Instead, turn it frequently—every minute is best. It'll cook just as fast, and you'll reduce the formation of those carcinogens.

And although I'm not a great fan of microwaves, briefly microwaving the meat before grilling actually removes some of the molecular building blocks of HCAs—sugars, creatinine, and some amino acids. All you need to do is shove it in the microwave for a "pretreatment" of 1½ to 2 minutes.

Another tip to make eating grilled meats safer: Load up with veggies. Eating cruciferous vegetables like broccoli along with grilled meats seems to change the way your body actually metabolizes the chemicals created in grilling. And use marinades. They serve as a protective wall against the heat, and because less fat drips onto the coals, they help to reduce the creation of HCAs.

Obviously the highest risk is associated with the highest consumption of well-done, charred, or blackened grilled meats, but as noted health writer Tara Parker Pope points out, we have no idea what the "safe" dose of either of these carcinogenic compounds is. For safety in grilling, she—and we—suggests following these basic guidelines:

1. Cook red meat rare or medium (If you use grass-fed beef, you minimize the risk of *E. coli* (see "Top Seven Reasons to Buy Grass-Fed Meat" on page 49), but just to be safe, always cook beef just past the point where it's pink.
2. Keep the temperature low, no matter what form of heat you use.
3. Gas grills may help because they give you more control of the cooking temperature.
4. If you don't have a gas grill, use wood chips made from hardwoods. They burn at a lower temperature than softwoods.
5. Use tongs. Forks puncture the meat and release juices, which can then splash down on the coals.

Baby Spinach Salad with Fresh Raspberries
Loaded with vitamin K for healthy bones

Prep Time: 5 to 10 minutes
Cook Time: None

Ingredients

6 cups (180 g) baby spinach

⅓ cup (50 g) crumbled feta cheese or
soft goat cheese

⅓ cup (33 g) sliced almonds, walnuts,
or pecans

1 cup (110 g) fresh raspberries

2 tablespoons (30 ml) raspberry
vinegar

2 tablespoons (40 g) seedless raspberry
jam, juice-sweetened

½ teaspoon seeded Dijon mustard

½ teaspoon raw honey or agave
nectar, to taste

In a large salad bowl, combine the spinach, cheese, nuts, and raspberries.

In a small bowl, whisk together the vinegar, jam, mustard, and honey or agave nectar. Drizzle the dressing over top of the salad and toss gently to coat. Serve immediately.

Yield: 4 servings

Suggested Swaps

- Roasted Red Pepper Dip and Crudités
  (page 146)

- Cranberry-Orange Relish
  (page 234)

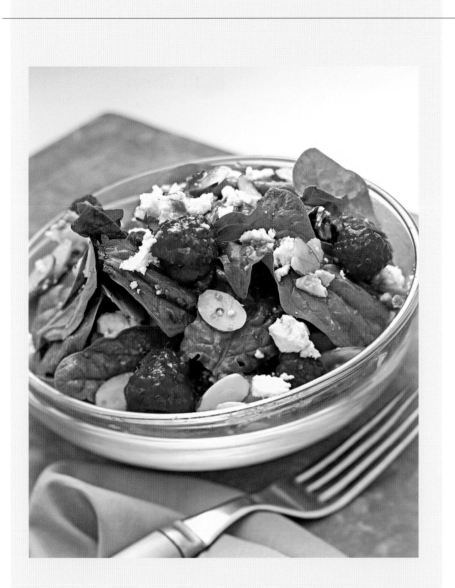

Notes from the Kitchen

- Unless it's triple washed, spinach is almost always gritty. To get rid of all dirt particles, fill your sink with water and gently agitate the leaves for a few minutes to allow the dirt to settle to the bottom. If you use a vegetable wash (a soapless cleanser designed to help remove wax, dirt, and agricultural chemicals from produce) in the water—even better! Store delicate washed leaves like spinach or lettuce with a moist paper towel to prolong freshness.

- Add some diced protein to this salad to make a nice summer meal.

- To add healthy fats, leave out ½ tablespoon of the vinegar and add 1 to 2 teaspoons flaxseed oil.

Broccoli Rabe with Raspberry-Vinegar Reduction

Packed with protective plant compounds

Prep Time: 5 minutes
Cook Time: 10 minutes

Ingredients

2 pounds (900 g) broccoli rabe

2 to 3 garlic scapes, stem chopped
   coarsely, bulb discarded (about
   ⅛ cup or 15 g) or 2 to 3 cloves garlic,
   minced, to taste

1 tablespoon (15 ml) olive oil

¼ teaspoon sea salt

½ teaspoon red-pepper flakes, optional

¼ cup (60 ml) vegetable or beef broth

3 tablespoons (45 ml) raspberry
   vinegar

Remove the tough stem ends from the rabe and chop the leaves and tender stems into 3-inch (8-cm) sections, leaving any small florets intact. Submerge the greens in a full sink of water and rinse well. Use a salad spinner to remove excess moisture.

In a 5- or 6-quart (5- or 6-L) sauté pan over medium heat, sauté the garlic in the oil for 1 minute. (Do not brown.) Add the broccoli rabe, salt, and red-pepper flakes and sauté for 2 to 3 minutes, or until wilted. Add the broth, cover, and steam until tender, for 3 to 5 minutes, turning over occasionally. Remove the broccoli to a serving dish and add the vinegar to the pan. Bring the liquid to a simmer and cook it down a bit, 1 to 2 minutes. Drizzle the liquid over the broccoli, toss, and serve.

Yield: 4 servings

Suggested Swaps

- Wild Rice and Green Beans with Shiitake Sauté (page 82)
- Sweet Beets and Greens (page 164)

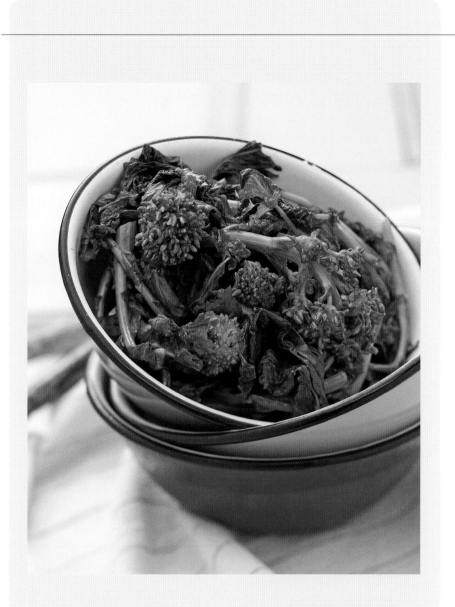

Notes from the Kitchen

- Freshness makes a big difference with broccoli rabe; it's best eaten shortly after harvest. It is naturally bitter, and the bitterness takes on a biting quality while the stems and leaves toughen if stored for too long.

- Garlic scapes are the immature stalks of the garlic plant before the bulb has fully developed. Most easily available in the early months of the growing season, they are green, tender, and mild tasting. They're the perfect accompaniment to all kinds of raw, wilted, or sautéed greens. You can snip them easily with scissors into desired sections and eat raw or lightly cooked.

- This salad combines three strong flavors into one dish: bitter (rabe), pungent (red-pepper flakes and garlic), and sour (vinegar).

- A salad spinner is a great, inexpensive piece of equipment to have in the kitchen. It's the best for drying fresh washed greens.

- Artisan vinegars are a key ingredient to dressing up plain foods simply and giving them a gourmet taste with little effort. A reduction makes a quick and easy tangy accompaniment to salads, vegetables, and meats. Noted researcher, nutritionist, and www.menshealth.com contributor Jeff Volek, Ph.D., R.D., suggests a salad with vinegar at the beginning of every meal for its potential help with managing blood sugar!

Real-Food Brownies

High-fiber and heart-healthy

Prep Time: 15 minutes
Cook Time: 45 minutes

Ingredients

1¼ cups (about 10 ounces, or 225 g)
   pitted dates

9 tablespoons (⅓ cup plus ¼ cup, or
   72 g) high-quality cacao or cocoa
   powder

¼ cup (60 ml) macadamia nut oil

½ cup (170 g) agave nectar

2 cups (450 g) canned garbanzo beans,
   rinsed and drained (one 28-ounce
   can works), or 2 cups (200 g) fresh
   cooked beans (see "Canned versus
   Dried Beans" on page 35)

4 eggs

½ teaspoon baking powder

1 teaspoon ground cinnamon

Preheat the oven to 350°F (180°C, gas mark 4).

Measure the dates into a liquid measuring cup and pour in hot water to the 1½ cup (355 ml) line, turning the dates over with your hands until the water reaches all the dates. Let sit for at least 10 minutes. Pour off ¼ cup (60 ml) of the liquid in the dates and process the rest in a blender or food processor until it forms a smooth paste.

Put the date paste into a large bowl and add the cacao or cocoa powder, oil, and agave nectar, mixing well.

Combine the beans and eggs in a blender or food processor and process until very smooth. Add the garbanzo mixture to the date mixture, stirring well to combine. Add the baking powder and cinnamon, stirring to combine, and pour the batter into a 9-inch (23-cm), nonstick pan or pie dish. (If using glass, you can grease lightly with a little oil or Natucol.)

Bake for 45 minutes. Cool for at least 15 minutes, cut, and serve. Store the remainder in the refrigerator.

Yield: 12 brownies

Suggested Swaps

• Silken Chocolate Parfaits (page 208)

• Baked Apples (page 188)

Notes from the Kitchen

- These brownies are not chewy, but they have a dense consistency closer to chocolate bread pudding or flourless chocolate cake. They're rich and satisfying and loaded with fiber.

- Medjool dates have a naturally high sugar content. The carbohydrate content is about half glucose and half fructose, plus some fiber. Date sugar is very coarse and doesn't dissolve easily, but if you use the entire (pitted) date instead of the extracted sugars, it actually works quite well as a sweetener for baked goods. The trick is to soak and soften the dates in a small amount of water first, and then blend them into a smooth paste in a food processor. Most of the time you can't even taste the date flavors; you just taste their delicious sweetness.

The Best Natural Sweeteners

Consumers have a lot of options when it comes to sweetening their food—here are our choices for the best natural ones on the market.

- Stevia is one of the few sweeteners that almost everyone agrees is a healthy choice. But for reasons only known to the bureaucratic powers-that-be, it's not allowed to be sold as a sweetener in the United States, and instead is classified as a "supplement." It's much sweeter than sugar, but has a slightly licorice-like aftertaste that not everyone loves. And it doesn't stand up well to heat. Other than that, stevia is a fine choice!

- We're big fans of xylitol, a sugar alcohol with a low glycemic index that actually has some health benefits in that it helps prevent bacteria from adhering to teeth and gums. You can buy xylitol in bulk from health food stores (or at www.jonnybowden.com). Unlike stevia, it stands up well to heat and mixes like sugar.

- Lo Han is fast building a reputation as one of the best natural sweeteners around. An extract of a fruit that's native to China, it's nearly 300 times sweeter than sugar and has about 2 calories per gram. Research suggests that it also works as an antioxidant and antiviral agent.

- Agave nectar is derived from the wild agave plant, a cactus-like plant native to Mexico that is best known for its role in making tequila. It's sweeter than sucrose and has a vanishingly low glycemic index. You can find it in most health food stores or supermarkets.

- Erythritol is a naturally derived sugar substitute that has been used in Japan since the early 1990s. It looks and tastes like sugar, has almost no calories, and has a glycemic index of zero. Not only that, it doesn't cause any digestive upset like some other sugar alcohols can do. And it doesn't contribute to tooth decay. The only downside? It's hard to find.

Remember, both raw organic honey and blackstrap molasses are also great sweeteners. Both are "real foods."

Chapter 2 **Pantry List**

FOOD GROUP	FOOD
Dairy	Cheese (crumbled feta or soft goat) Eggs
Herbs/Spices/ Condiments	Cinnamon Dijon mustard (seeded) Garlic Peppercorns (red or black) Raspberry jam (seedless), juice-sweetened Raw sugar Red pepper flakes Sea salt
Meat	Sirloin steaks
Miscellaneous	Agave nectar (or raw honey) Baking powder Broth (vegetable or beef) Cacao or cocoa powder Garbanzo beans (canned or fresh) Macadamia nut oil Olive oil, extra virgin Red wine, dry Vinegar (raspberry) Vegetable oil, (such as avocado)
Nuts/Seeds	Almonds (or walnuts or pecans)
Produce	Baby spinach Broccoli rabe Dates (pitted) Mushrooms (dried) Onions (green) Raspberries

Clockwise from top left:
Broiled Salmon with Tamari-Orange
Marinade, Dandelion Greens with
Warm Sesame Dressing, Spiced Pear
Sorbet, Wild Rice and Green Beans
with Shiitake Sauté

CHAPTER 3

Omega Star

Broiled Salmon with Tamari-Orange Marinade

MEAL:

80 Broiled Salmon with Tamari-Orange Marinade

82 Wild Rice and Green Beans with Shiitake Sauté

84 Dandelion Greens with Warm Sesame Dressing

86 Spiced Pear Sorbet

AH, THE '80s.

In case you've mercifully forgotten them, it was a time when MTV played music videos by Haircut 100, Tom Cruise was synonymous with *Risky Business*, people played Pong, and "must-see TV" meant *The Cosby Show*.

And good nutrition meant "low fat."

But that was then. Today, most people understand that all fat isn't bad. And the "poster food" for everything that's good about fat is salmon.

SALMON: HEALTHY FATS FROM THE SEA

According to the U.S. National Fisheries Institute, the per capita consumption of salmon in America went from less than a pound a year in 1992 to more than 2 pounds a year in 2006. And that's only an average. Among health-conscious Americans it's not unusual to eat salmon weekly—or even more frequently. The reason? Salmon is loaded with two of the healthiest fats on the planet: the omega-3 fatty acids known as DHA (docosahexaenoic acid) and EPA (eicosapentaenoic acid). And it's absolutely delicious here in **Broiled Salmon with Tamari-Orange Marinade**.

Essential fatty acids were discovered in the early 1930s by husband-and-wife medical team George and Marilyn Burr. The Burrs found that rats deprived of fat developed a number of metabolic disturbances and symptoms, including scaly skin, growth retardation, and reproductive problems. Once fat was reintroduced into the rats' diet, most of these problems disappeared. This led to the discovery of essential fatty acids, which are fats that are essential for health and that the body can't actually make on its own—they need to be obtained in the diet.

Even though the two fatty acids in salmon, DHA and EPA, are among the most important compounds in human nutrition, they're not technically essential fatty acids. Why? Because the body actually can make them from another omega-3 fatty acid called alpha-linolenic acid, which is essential. But what the body can do and what it actually does do are two different things. Even if you're taking in plenty of alpha-linolenic acid from flaxseed (which most people aren't doing to begin with), very little of the alpha-linolenic acid actually converts to DHA and EPA, so you wind up noticeably lacking in these two incredibly important nutrients. And that's not a good thing at all.

This is especially tragic because it's so simple to get enough DHA and EPA. They're packaged together in one tidy food: salmon. DHA and EPA work together brilliantly. And their combined benefits to your health are beyond stunning. Hundreds of studies show that the omega-3 fatty acids found in salmon benefit the heart and the brain, improving both mood and behavior.

How to Cook Salmon

Probably the most important thing to remember when cooking fish is that it will continue to cook after it is off the heat, so you have to remove it before it is done to your liking. As the fish is cooking, cut into it frequently with a fork and look inside to check for doneness.

While most fish taste best when they flake and are opaque, this is not the case with salmon, which tastes best when it's on the rare side. So when you're cooking, look for the center to still be translucent. As a general guideline, grill salmon for 7 to 8 minutes per each inch (3 cm) of thickness.

Because of the wonderful healthy fat content of salmon, it does well in many cooking styles, including grilling, baking, poaching, broiling, and pan-frying. Crazy as it sounds, some people poach salmon in their dishwashers!

DHA DELIVERS

The first of these two omega-3 fatty acids, DHA, is brain food and is crucial for vision. It's the most abundant fat in the brain and the retina, and it is vitally important during pregnancy, where it's linked to the development of the baby's brain and eyes. DHA is also an important component of breast milk, and it's well documented that breast-fed infants and toddlers score better on cognitive and visual tests, perhaps because of the DHA. Both the World Health Organization and the British Nutrition Foundation recommend that infant formula be supplemented with DHA. And in a 2002 study of almost 9,000 pregnant women published in the *British Medical Journal*, researchers found that the babies of women who ate fish once a week during their first trimesters had more than 3½ times less risk of low birth weight and premature birth.

DHA isn't just important for babies. In 1998, scientists at the Agricultural Research Service of the USDA found that volunteers who ate foods enriched with DHA showed an increase in HDL cholesterol (the protective kind) and lowered their triglycerides by 26 percent.

EPA ESSENTIALS

EPA, the other important omega-3 fatty acid found in salmon, has complementary benefits. The March 2007 edition of the journal *Atherosclerosis* published a study in which some Japanese men with unhealthy blood sugar levels were given 1,800 mg a day of EPA for approximately 2 years. The men had a significant decrease in the thickness of their carotid arteries along with an improvement of blood flow.

Another study, this one published in the medical journal *The Lancet* (also March 2007), showed that people with high cholesterol levels who were on statin drugs reduced their frequency of major cardio events by almost 20 percent when they added EPA supplements to their daily regimens.

THE POWER OF THE PAIR

DHA and EPA are known to be mood enhancers. They incorporate themselves into cell membranes, making the membranes more fluid and making it easier for important brain chemicals such as dopamine and serotonin to get in and out. They help the brain to repair damage. Both DHA and EPA together are being studied in ongoing research at Harvard University by Andrew Stoll, M.D., for their effect on the depression of bipolar disorder. Also, a University of Pittsburgh study showed that the omega-3 fatty acids found in fatty fish such as salmon are associated with increased gray matter volume in areas of the brain commonly linked to mood and behavior.

A ton of studies link low omega-3 consumption to depression, mood disorders, and behavioral problems, including those that are especially worrisome among kids and teenagers, such as violence, acting out, and possibly ADHD. Research by Sarah Conklin, Ph.D., at the Cardiovascular Behavioral Medicine Program in the department of psychiatry at the University of Pittsburgh, reported that people who had lower blood levels of omega-3 fatty acids were more likely to have negative outlooks and to be more impulsive. And in 2001, Joseph Hibbeln, M.D., a senior investigator at the National Institutes of Health, published a study that found a correlation between a higher intake of omega-3 fatty acids (mostly from fish) and lower murder rates!

Another way that omega-3 fatty acids provide health benefits is by reducing inflammation. Chronic, low-grade inflammation is emerging as a major risk factor for a host of chronic diseases, so much so that it was dubbed the "silent killer" in a *Time* magazine cover story a few years ago. Inflammation contributes to obesity, diabetes, cancer, Alzheimer's disease, arthritis, and probably some conditions we haven't even thought of yet. And the omega-3s are among the most anti-inflammatory compounds in the world. A diet filled with natural anti-inflammatories (such as the omega-3 fatty acids found in salmon and flaxseeds and the many anti-inflammatory compounds found in the vegetables featured in this book) is one of the best preventive health strategies you could possibly follow.

EPA and DHA: What the Experts Recommend

The World Health Organization and the North Atlantic Treaty Organization (WHO-NATO) recommend consuming 0.3 to 0.5 g a day of EPA and DHA.

The 2005 Dietary Guidelines Advisory Committee recommends consuming two 4-ounce (115 g) servings of fish high in EPA and DHA per week (such as salmon) to reduce the risk of coronary heart disease.

The American Heart Association recommends 0.5 to 1.8 g per day of EPA and DHA to reduce the risk of cardiac disease, plus 1.5 to 3 g of alpha-linolenic acid, which is found in flaxseeds and flaxseed oil, for even more benefit.

How to Poach Fruit

Poached fruit—which is simply fruit cooked in simmering liquid—is a wonderful, simple, healthy dessert.

It is best to use firm, ripe fruit. But poaching is also a great use for out-of-season or underripe fruit that is too hard eat on its own. You can poach practically any fruit, but the most common are pears, peaches, and apples.

You can poach fruit in pretty much any sweetened liquid, such as water, juice, or wine. One example is 2 cups (475 ml) water and ⅓ cup (113 g) honey. The liquid has to be sweet, or else the poaching will pull the fruit's natural sugars out. For example, pears are often poached in sweetened red wine, which gives the fruit a rich flavor and a beautiful, deep ruby color.

If you wish, you can spice up the flavor of poached fruit by adding flavorings such as cloves, cinnamon, or vanilla to the liquid.

Poaching times vary greatly, from a few minutes to more than a half hour, depending on the size and firmness of the fruit. For example, apples and pears take up to 35 minutes. As you're poaching fruit, test it frequently by piercing it with the tip of a knife. Cook until you are satisfied with the tenderness of the fruit. Take the pan off of the heat, but let the fruit cool right in the poaching liquid. Once the fruit has cooled, remove it with a slotted spoon and carefully scoop out the core, if necessary, with a paring knife.

Experiment with different types of fruit, poaching liquids, and seasonings. Here's one combination to try:

6 pears
2 bottles red wine
1 cup (340 g) honey
1 split vanilla bean
and 2 cinnamon sticks.

The omega-3s in fish are among the most heart-healthy nutrients on the planet. Even the FDA gave them a "qualified health claim" in September of 2006, stating that "supportive but not conclusive research shows that the consumption of EPA and DHA omega-3 fatty acids may reduce the risk of coronary heart disease." Don't be fooled by the FDA's overly cautious language. Fish such as salmon is a big component of nearly every native diet that has been shown to be associated with lower rates of heart disease. According to Stoll, omega-3s reduce the rate of fatal arrhythmias by 30 percent. "In the United States alone, more than 70,000 lives could be saved each year if Americans had sufficient omega-3s in their bodies," he says.

We don't.

Most of us get a paltry 0.1 to 0.2 g a day of EPA and DHA (that's one-tenth to two-tenths of a gram!). (For what health organizations advise, see "EPA and DHA: What the Experts Recommend" on page 71.)

Personally, I'd like to see us get a minimum of 0.5 g a day of EPA and DHA, and ideally 1 to 3 g. You can meet the World Health Organization and the North Atlantic Treaty Organization (WHO-NATO) recommendations by consuming 2 servings of salmon (or other fatty fish such as mackerel) each week.

And if all this hasn't convinced you of the incredible health benefits of frequent meals of salmon, let me appeal to your vanity. Salmon can make you look better. Nicholas Perricone, M.D., whose books on skin care have topped the best-seller list on numerous occasions, recommends a "three-day diet" for clearing up your skin that features—what else—salmon. For breakfast even! (Hey, it's not that weird to the folks fishing through the ice in Greenland!) Actually, Perricone's "three-day nutritional face-lift" claims to give your skin the same results that a face-lift would, by eating salmon two or three times a day, accompanied by fresh fruits and vegetables. I can't guarantee that, but I'm pretty sure you'd look and feel pretty terrific after allowing your skin and hair cells to be bathed in the nectar of those nourishing omega-3s.

Salmon: Wild versus Farm Raised

In this great debate, I'm strongly on the side of wild salmon. Here's why: Farm-raised salmon are the fish equivalent of factory-farmed animals. Much like factory-farmed animals, farm-raised salmon are raised in confined quarters (essentially saltwater feedlots) that often promote ill health and have to be controlled by the widespread use of antibiotics and/or pesticides. According to the Coastal Alliance for Aquaculture Reform, farmed salmon are fed more antibiotics per pound of body weight than any livestock animal in North America.

To make matters worse, although some fisheries feed their salmon ground-up versions of the fish they might normally feed on, many farm-raised salmon are fed grains, which is not their natural diet. Because of this, farm-raised salmon have much less omega-3 fats in their bodies than wild salmon.

Also, farm-raised salmon have much higher levels of cancer-causing PCBs than their wild brethren. By some reports, they also contain other highly toxic pesticides. And U.S. investigators recently found that farm-raised salmon have been eating fish meal laced with the same chemical linked to a recent pet food recall: melamine.

Even more bad news: While wild salmon get their red color from dining on krill and ingesting a natural antioxidant carotenoid called astaxanthin, farmed salmon often get their color from pigments and colorings added to their naturally gray flesh.

On the other hand, wild Alaskan salmon are among the purest of all ocean species. Residing in remote and pristine waters, they're small fish that feed at the lower end of the food chain. And wild Alaskan salmon, including the sockeye salmon, are grown in sustainable fisheries free of antibiotics, pesticides, coloring agents, and growth hormones.

When my book *The 150 Healthiest Foods on Earth* came out, I received a number of letters from scientists working for factory-farmed salmon companies. For the most part, these were sincere, knowledgeable people who assured me that I was wrong about the dangers of farm-raised salmon. While each could only speak about their own fisheries, they assured me that, at least in their operations, great care was taken in the raising of these fish, that their contamination levels were very low, and that their fish contained plenty of omega-3 fats. Some of the scientists pointed out that I might be doing a disservice scaring people away from one of the healthiest foods on earth and that farm-raised salmon was certainly better than no salmon at all.

While I remain unconvinced, I'm willing to grant that some farm operations are caring and careful and produce a decent product. The problem is knowing which ones they are. In general, I stand by my position that wild salmon from reputable, reliable sources is best. When at all possible, I'd stick with the wild kind. My personal recommendation is salmon from Vital Choice seafood, a small company with more than fifty years of experience harvesting Alaskan salmon. It's run by dedicated fishermen who are committed to sustainable fishing and an absolutely pure product. You can find them online or through a link on my website www.jonnybowden.com under "Shopping" then "Healthy Foods."

DANDELION GREENS: MORE THAN JUST WEEDS

Besides the delicious, nutritious salmon, another highlight of this meal is a food that most people in America consider a weed: dandelion greens. You'll love it in **Dandelion Greens with Warm Sesame Dressing**.

It may surprise you to find out that dandelions rank among the top four green vegetables in terms of their overall nutritional value. Dandelion greens are used in healing traditions around the world, and its Latin name—*taraxacum officinale*—actually means "official remedy for the disorders."

Probably at the top of the list of things dandelion is good for is helping the liver to do its job of detoxifying. It's no wonder that you'll see dandelion tea touted on self-help hepatitis websites.

Dandelion also contains inulin, which is a naturally occurring soluble fiber that's known to have a positive effect on blood sugar levels. Dandelion is also one of the best greens for PMS, and it is a great natural diuretic that can help with water retention and bloat. Dandelion stimulates the digestive organs and helps prompt the liver and gallbladder to release bile, which can help with constipation and indigestion. And a 1-cup (20-g) serving of dandelion also contains a respectable 3 g of fiber, all for a ridiculously low 35 calories!

Bear in mind that dandelion greens have a strong and bitter taste, and so they need a flavor counterpoint to make them palatable. But once you taste them in our amazing sauce—which is made with raw honey, macadamia nut oil, and spicy Asian mustard—you'll never think of dandelion greens as inedible weeds again. This side dish also contains some sesame seeds, which are rich in plant chemicals of the lignan family that, at least in animal studies, have been shown to enhance fat burning.

Rice adds a nice texture and flavor to the meal, and it's smashing in **Wild Rice and Green Beans with Shiitake Sauté**. While it's no nutritional heavyweight, wild rice still provides 3 g of fiber per cup and a few minerals to boot. And it's easy on the digestive system.

A SORBET A DAY...

Then there's that **Spiced Pear Sorbet**. It's a great alternative to ice cream. "Why do I need an alternative?" you may be wondering. "I'm doing just fine with my Ben and Jerry's." Well, believe me, I understand. (More than you might suspect, unfortunately!) Ice cream is fine in its place (especially my favorite, the goat's milk kind), but most of the ice cream we buy is terrible, loaded with sugar, calories, emulsifiers, and a baker's dozen unpronounceable chemicals and artificial flavors.

The Spiced Pear Sorbet, on the other hand, has far fewer calories and sugar, and its taste comes from the pear itself, plus a few delicious natural spices, not artificial flavors. And one medium pear comes direct from the pear tree with 5 g of fiber (more than a tablespoon of Metamucil powder!), plus a dollop of potassium, a smattering of minerals, and 13 mg of phytosterols, a class of plant chemicals that are known to have a myriad of health benefits. Plus a pear provides you with a little taste of the new superstars of eye nutrition, antioxidants lutein and zeaxanthin.

Need one more reason to love pears? According to the results of the Iowa Women's Health study, which tracked the dietary habits of nearly 35,000 women over a fifteen year period, pears were one of the few foods associated with reduced coronary heart disease and cardiovascular disease mortality.

Enjoy!

Meal Prep Tips

- Spiced Pear Sorbet should be prepared ahead of time. Its preparation is a two-step process: stewing the pears and freezing them, then pureeing the frozen pears with the other ingredients. Both steps can be completed up to a week before the meal, or you can complete step two the day of the meal.

- Prepare the marinade 4 to 6 hours ahead to allow the salmon time to soak up the flavors.

- Start the meal by preparing the Wild Rice and Green Beans with Shiitake Sauté.

- When the beans are set at a simmer, remove the salmon and let it rest for about 30 minutes.

- Prepare the Dandelion Greens with Warm Sesame Dressing while the beans are cooking, and broil the salmon last.

- Both the beans and greens dishes will yield extra portions. Store them in the fridge to enjoy over the next one to three days.

- Soften the Spiced Pear Sorbet at room temperature for 10 to 15 minutes before serving.

Broiled Salmon with Tamari-Orange Marinade

Full of omega-3s for your heart, mood, and skin

Prep Time: 10 minutes, then marinate for 4 to 6 hours
Cook Time: 10 to 15 minutes

Ingredients

1½ pounds (680 g) wild Alaskan salmon fillet, cut into 4 equal portions, or four 6-ounce (186-g) salmon steaks

⅓ cup (80 ml) high-quality dry white wine, such as Chardonnay, or medium sweet wine, such as Riesling

2 tablespoons (30 ml) low-sodium tamari

⅓ cup (80 ml) orange juice (fresh squeezed is best; about 1 large juicy orange)

3 tablespoons (24 g) peeled and finely grated ginger

¼ cup (25 g) finely chopped green onions

1 teaspoon raw honey

½ teaspoon extra virgin olive oil

Rinse the salmon gently in water and pat to dry.

In a small bowl, combine the wine, tamari, orange juice, ginger, scallions, and honey and whisk to combine well.

Place the salmon in a shallow glass baking pan, skin side down if fillet, and pour the marinade evenly on top.

Cover the baking pan with plastic wrap and refrigerate for 4 to 6 hours or overnight, tipping the dish occasionally to recoat the salmon.

Remove the baking pan from the refrigerator and let it stand at room temperature for 30 minutes. Preheat the broiler.

Lift the salmon out of the baking pan and remove any ginger or scallions to prevent burning. Rub the oil on the skin/bottom side of the salmon and place it on the broiling pan, oiled side down.

Broil the salmon under high heat for 10 to 15 minutes, until the salmon flakes easily with a fork and the flesh inside is firm and light pink. The top should lightly brown and caramelize. (If the salmon browns within the first 5 minutes, move the broiling pan down 1 rack in your oven.)

Yield: 4 servings

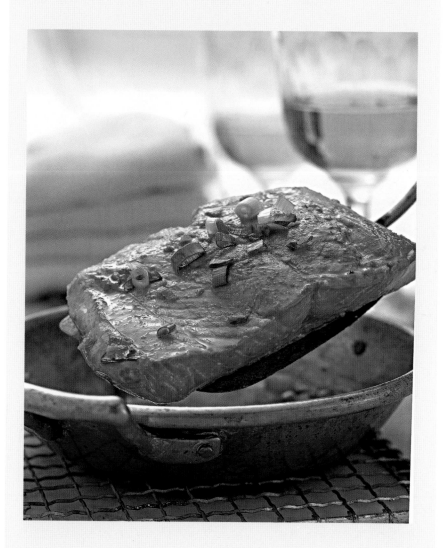

Notes from the Kitchen

- Marinades impart wonderful flavors to proteins—such as meat, fish, and tofu—and the acid and salt components of the marinade can help to tenderize the meat or fish. It takes time for the protein to fully absorb the marinade flavors. Seafood takes the least, 4 hours, whereas heavier cuts of meat take longer, up to 12 hours. A typical marinade combines a strongly flavored liquid—such as wine, vinegar, or juice—with herbs, spices, or other flavoring foods, such as minced onion, and a small amount of oil. You can omit the oil to reduce the fat content. Using a small amount of a pungent-flavored food or spice such as garlic, cayenne pepper, or ginger will reduce the need for salt.

- One cup of marinade is sufficient for 2 to 3 pounds (900 g to 1¼ kg) of protein.

- It's helpful to turn the meat, seafood, or tofu to recoat it occasionally while marinating. Some people combine the meat, seafood, or tofu and marinade in a gallon-size resealable plastic bag to easily recoat the meat. Place the bag inside a bowl in the refrigerator just in case the bag leaks.

Wild Rice and Green Beans with Shiitake Sauté
Full of fiber and minerals

Prep Time: 10 minutes
Cook Time: 50 minutes to 1 hour

Ingredients

½ cup (80 g) dry wild rice

4 cups (940 ml) water or no-sodium added chicken or vegetable broth

¼ teaspoon sea salt, omit if using broth

12 ounces (336 g) fresh green beans (about 3 cups), ends removed

2 tablespoons (28 g) butter

1 tablespoon (15 ml) extra virgin olive oil

2 shallots, finely chopped

2 cups (140 g) fresh shiitake mushrooms, stems removed and caps cut into strips

¼ cup (60 ml) rice wine, sake, or white wine

In a large saucepan with a tightly fitting lid, place the rice and water or broth.

Bring to a boil, stir, reduce the heat, and simmer for 40 minutes. Add the salt, if using, and green beans, and continue to boil for 10 to 15 minutes longer, or until the beans are tender-crisp. Remove from the heat and let rest, covered, for 5 minutes. Strain off any remaining liquid.

In a sauté pan over medium heat, heat the butter and oil until the butter melts. Add the shallots and sauté for 2 minutes. Add the mushrooms and toss to coat, sautéing until tender, about 4 minutes. Add the wine or sake and sauté for an additional 2 minutes, until most of the liquid is absorbed or evaporated. Add the green bean and rice mixture and serve immediately.

Yield: 8 servings

If you prefer, omit the green beans, increase the rice to 1 cup (160 g), and decrease the water to 3 cups (705 ml).

Suggested Swaps

- Confetti Basmati Rice (page 36)
- Steam-Baked Vidalia Onions (page 104)

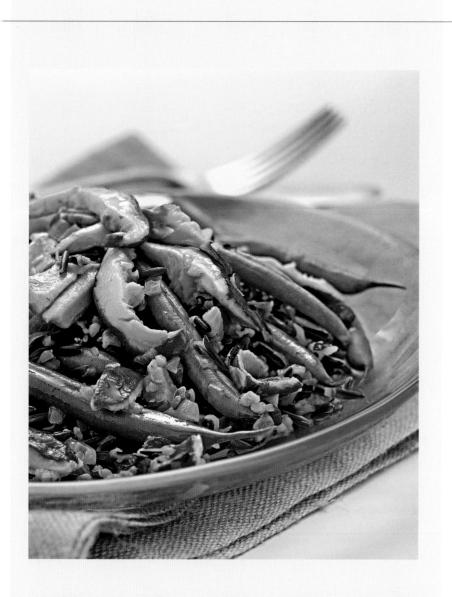

Notes from the Kitchen

- Wild rice cooks more like pasta than other rices: It will not absorb all the water, so the liquid measurement doesn't need to be exact.

- Hand-harvested natural wild rice cooks more quickly than farmed wild rice: about 30 minutes total cooking time versus 40 to 55 minutes.

- Rice is done when it just puffs open. Do not overcook rice, or it will become mushy. Shorter cooking time yields a chewier texture.

- This shallot and mushroom sauté is also delicious over lean cuts of beef or marinated baked tofu.

- Try switching out the mushroom and wine varieties for different flavor bases.

Dandelion Greens with Warm Sesame Dressing

Liver and digestive system support

Prep Time: 5 to 10 minutes
Cook Time: 4 minutes

Ingredients

6 cups (360 g) fresh dandelion greens
(about 1 pound)

2 tablespoons (30 ml) brown (or any)
rice vinegar

2 teaspoons (13 g) raw honey or
agave nectar

1 tablespoon (15 g) spicy Asian
mustard or seedless Dijon mustard

1 tablespoon (15 ml) macadamia nut oil

¼ cup (30 g) sesame seeds

Wash the greens and spin to dry. Remove and discard the long stems and chop or tear the greens into bite-size pieces, placing them in a large salad bowl.

In a small bowl, combine the vinegar, honey or agave nectar, and mustard and set aside.

In a small skillet over medium-low heat, heat the oil until hot but not smoking. Add the vinegar mixture and cook, stirring regularly, for about 1 minute. Add the sesame seeds and cook, continuing to stir, for 1 to 2 minutes. Spoon over the greens, toss well, and serve immediately.

Yield: 6 servings

Suggested Swaps

• Asparagus-Endive Salad (page 206)

• Haricot Verts with Pomegranate Mint
  (page 186)

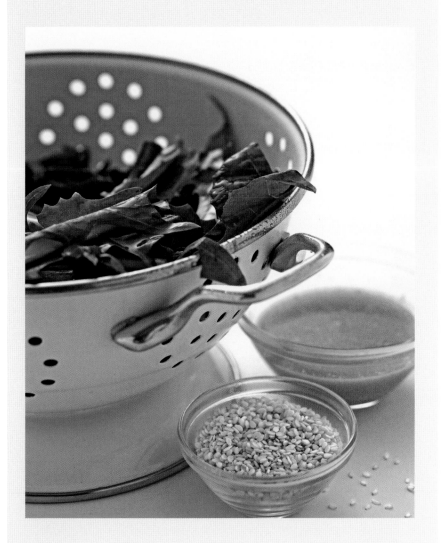

Notes from the Kitchen

- For a less Asian feel, change the types of vinegar, mustard, and nuts. For instance, try using balsamic vinegar, Dijon mustard, and chopped pecans.

- You can usually buy dandelion greens at large grocery stores. When we tested this dish, however, we couldn't find any dandelion greens in the markets. So we weeded our yards, picking about 8 cups (480 g) of young dandelion leaves. They were shorter and more bitter than what you tend to find at the grocery store, but the dressing worked beautifully even with their extra-strong, wild flavor. If you pick wild dandelions, be sure you know exactly what you're picking and eating. Never, ever pick dandelions that could have been exposed to pesticides. If you're not sure, don't take a chance.

- Hot dressings will partially cook the tender leaves of a salad. This is a perfect technique for wilting and mellowing the tougher or more bitter varieties of salad greens.

- Unlike most dressed salads, this dish also tastes good cold next day. The greens will be sweeter and softer.

Spiced Pear Sorbet

Antioxidant ally

Prep Time: 15 minutes, 1 hour for chilling, and 5 hours for freezing
Cook Time: 10 to 20 minutes

Ingredients

2 pounds (900 g) ripe
  Anjou pears (4 medium)

½ cup (120 ml) pear juice, apple cider,
  or water, more if pears are not fully
  ripe, plus ⅓ cup (80 ml) for processing

1 to 2 tablespoons (15 to 28 ml) ginger
  juice (see "Notes from the Kitchen")

7 whole cloves, optional

2 to 3 tablespoons (12 to 18 g)
  crystallized ginger, optional

¼ teaspoon vanilla extract

Peel and core the pears. Halve and quarter them, then cut the quarters in half through the middle.

In a medium saucepan, place the pears; pear juice, cider, or water; ginger juice; and cloves, if using. Bring to a rapid boil over medium-high heat, stir, cover, and reduce the heat. Simmer, covered, for 10 to 20 minutes, until the pears are very soft. (The riper the pears, the faster they'll cook.)

Transfer the pears and sauce to a stainless steel bowl, cover with waxed paper, and cool in the refrigerator for 1 hour to overnight.

Remove the condensation moisture from the waxed paper, recover, and transfer to the freezer for 5 hours to overnight.

Remove the bowl from the freezer and let thaw for 15 minutes. Run warm water under the bowl to thaw the bottom, if necessary.

Meanwhile, process the ginger in the food processor until pebble-size. Remove to a dish.

Remove the pears from the bowl and cut them with a heavy knife into smaller pieces to fit into the food processor, adding additional juice if necessary. Process the pears in small batches in the food processor until a creamy consistency is achieved. Stir in the ginger and vanilla and serve.

Freeze the remainder in a tightly covered container. Thaw at room temperature for about 15 minutes and stir well before serving.

Yield: 8 to 10 servings

Suggested Swaps

• Grilled Pineapple (page 148)

• Sweet and Simple Almond Butter
  Apricot Cookies (page 168)

Notes from the Kitchen

- To make ginger juice, peel and grate fresh ginger, then squeeze the juice out of the gratings. You'll need about 2 tablespoons (16 g) of gratings to get 1 tablespoon (15 ml) of juice.

- It's helpful to use a stainless steel bowl to make this sorbet for two reasons: First, stainless steel, like glass but unlike some plastics, never transfers odors or flavors from one dish to the next, even in the freezer. Second, it's easier to thaw the sorbet slightly (to get it out) with hot water over a thin steel bowl than a different type of container.

- Sorbets are great alternatives to ice cream. They can be prepared in advance and stored in airtight containers for a week or two.

- When making frozen fruit sorbets, you can eliminate the cooking step and save time by working with fresh berries. If a sweetener is required, try using agave nectar or raw honey.

- Cloves are an additional warmer for winter months; they may be omitted if you prefer less spicy flavor.

Five Foods to Fight Asthma

Research has shown the following foods—which we include in this book—can help you win the fight against asthma.

1. **Salmon.** The omega-3 fats in salmon (and other cold water fish) are anti-inflammatory. So are the omega-3's in flaxseeds. Asthmatics will benefit by having more anti-inflammatory compounds in their diet. Wild salmon fits the bill, as do sardines.

2. **Spinach and kale.** People with asthma tend to have lower levels of magnesium, and these foods are magnesium heavyweights. By one survey, more than 70 percent of Americans don't get the optimal amount of magnesium in their diet. Magnesium relaxes muscles (think Epson salts!) and may relax the upper respiratory muscles that tend to spasm in asthma.

3. **Red peppers.** They're high in vitamin C, which is particularly helpful in reducing the symptoms of exercise-induced asthma. According to Alan Gaby, M.D., vitamin C (ascorbic acid) inhibits production of an enzyme called phosphodiesterase, which is how many asthma drugs work. And red peppers are also high in vitamin A, which is often low in people who suffer from asthma attacks.

4. **Chinese cabbage.** This vegetable is a great source of vitamin B6, which appears to help correct abnormalities in metabolism frequently found in asthmatics. Stress is a big trigger for asthma, and vitamin B6 is a great stress-buster. Brewer's yeast, bananas, garbanzo beans, and chicken are other good sources.

5. **Onions.** This root vegetable is another great source of anti-inflammatory properties, particularly the wonderful flavonoid quercetin, which has anti-allergic properties as well. According to Gaby, onions also contain compounds that relax the bronchial passageways. (Caution: Raw and pickled onions may provoke asthma attacks in a small number of sensitive people, according to personal chef and food coach Lisa Turner.)

Chapter 3 **Pantry List**

FOOD GROUP	FOOD
Dairy	Butter
Grains	Wild Rice
Herbs/Spices/Condiments	Cloves Ginger (fresh) Ginger (crystallized) Ginger juice Honey (raw) Mustard (spicy Asian or seedless Dijon) Sea salt Vanilla extract
Miscellaneous	Broth (chicken or vegetable) Brown rice vinegar Macadamia nut oil Olive oil (extra virgin) Rice wine (or sake or white wine) Tamari White wine (dry or medium sweet)
Nuts/Seeds	Sesame seeds
Produce	Dandelion greens Green beans (fresh) Onions (green) Orange juice (fresh squeezed is best) Pears (Anjou) Pear juice (or apple cider) Shallots Shiitake mushrooms
Seafood	Wild Alaskan salmon fillet

Clockwise from top left:
Delicious Dal, Steam-Baked Vidalia
Onions, Raw Chocolate Fondue, Curried
Quinoa Greens with Coconut Dressing

CHAPTER 4

Anti-Inflammatory Immune-System Booster

Delicious Dal with Sweet Onion and Curried Greens

MEAL:

102 Delicious Dal with Sweet Onion and Curried Greens

104 Steam-Baked Vidalia Onions (with thanks to Andrew Rubman, N.D.)

106 Curried Quinoa Greens with Coconut Dressing

108 Raw Chocolate Fondue

THIS NUTRITIOUS AND DELICIOUS meal contains so many special delights that I almost don't know where to start. (Of course, I want to start with the raw chocolate fondue—how can you not—but I'll resist the temptation, especially since I told you all about the health benefits of cocoa in an earlier chapter.)

So let's start with the spices.

You may remember from elementary school history that spices were a big part of the commerce of ancient civilizations. The spice trade from India attracted the attention of both the Ptolemaic dynasty and the Roman Empire. The Romans sailed to Arabia and India to buy spices and incense. Later, from the early fifteenth century into the early seventeenth century, European ships traveled around the world in search of gold, silver, and ... spices. Vasco da Gama sacrificed three months without seeing land and the lives of two-thirds of the men he left with all in the service of finding another sea route to India. And a Dutch convoy that sailed to India in 1598 returned a year later with no less than 600,000 pounds of spices. To this day, India produces 1,600,000 tons of spices, 86 percent of the world spice production. (No other country is even close; the second biggest producer is China with 4 percent of the world's total.)

TURMERIC FOR TASTE AND HEALTH

As it turns out, all those explorers were on to something. Spices (and herbs) have been used for centuries for medicinal purposes, not to mention their awesome tastes. A good spice rack is a virtual medicine cabinet. Spices can help treat digestive disorders, lower blood sugar, reduce inflammation, fight free radicals, and even boost the metabolism. The spices in this meal are a superb group. And the entrée features what is arguably the most powerful spice in the world—turmeric.

Turmeric is part of the healing systems of India, China, and the Polynesian Islands, and it occupies a place of distinction in both Ayurvedic and Chinese medicine. The reason? Its phenomenal anti-inflammatory properties, which are due to the presence of compounds called curcuminoids, the most famous of which is curcumin. Curcumin is responsible for giving curry its trademark bright yellow color. Because of the anti-inflammatory actions of the curcuminoids, turmeric is traditionally used to treat arthritis. It also has significant cancer-fighting ability. At least thirty published animal studies show that curcumin either reduces the number of tumors, the size of tumors, or the percentage of animals that developed them. One study shows that turmeric inhibits the growth of human colon cancer cells.

And turmeric is one of the most liver-friendly foods on earth. Many holistic health practitioners use it to treat hepatitis C and other ailments when the liver needs nutritional support. Deepak Chopra, M.D., says that turmeric's "traditional purifying effect makes it a useful spice for people participating in a detoxification program." Curry powder, which is used in the side dish **Curried Quinoa Greens with Coconut Dressing**, also contains curcumin, so you get a nice double dose in this wonderful meal.

Another of the spices you'll find in this meal is cumin, an important medicinal herb in many African, Asian, and Arabian nations. In four different studies using the oil from black cumin seeds, people reported significantly fewer allergic symptoms. One study even found that the oil was effective in inactivating certain types of breast cancer cells, at least in a test tube. And according to Chopra, cumin can help reduce heartburn and improve digestion.

Cilantro, also called Chinese parsley, has a long and noble history as a digestive aid. (For you trivia buffs, the leaves of the plant are called cilantro while the seeds are called coriander.) The seeds have been rumored to be found in the tombs of the pharaohs, where they were placed to prevent indigestion in the afterlife. In the traditions of Qi-Gong—a form of Chinese energy medicine—cilantro is considered a highly detoxifying herb.

MAIN DISH MERITS

The main dish, **Delicious Dal**, actually combines the best of two worlds—the health benefits of lentils and curry. (By the way, for those who plan on being on Jeopardy!, the difference between lentils and beans is that lentils don't contain sulfur and therefore don't produce gas.) Lentils, like beans, are absolutely loaded with fiber, especially the soluble kind, which helps control blood sugar by delaying the emptying of the stomach and retarding the entry of sugar into the bloodstream. (See "What's Up with Fiber?" on page 110.) One cup (225 g) of lentils has a whopping 16 g of the stuff. High-fiber diets have consistently been associated with better glucose control for people with and without diabetes, not to mention better control of weight. High-fiber diets are also associated with a lower risk for both cancer and heart disease. And 1 cup (225 g) of lentils contains about 18 g of protein, which is about the same amount as a small protein shake.

You'll notice that the lentils are cooked in ghee. Ghee is actually clarified butter, and it occupies an almost sacred place as a healing food in the ancient system of Indian healing known as Ayurvedic medicine. My friend Dharm Singh Khalsa, M.D., author of *Food as Medicine*, reports that ghee is a highly regarded food in nutritional medicine. In Ayurvedic medicine, it's believed to help stimulate the flow of fluids through the body, rejuvenating the nervous system. My colleague Annemarie Colbin, author of *Food and Healing*, says ghee is one of the three best fats in the world to use for cooking. And remember, too, that in India, where ghee is used all the time, there are no "factory farms" for cows, so all animal products such as butter (or ghee) come from grass-fed animals. (See "Top Seven Reasons to Buy Grass-Fed Meat" on page 49 for more on grass-fed animals.)

KALE: BLUEBERRIES OF THE VEGETABLE KINGDOM

And then there's kale. I like to call kale the blueberries of the vegetable kingdom. Why? Because both these plant foods consistently score at the top of their categories in tests of antioxidant power. By one version of the ORAC (oxygen radical absorbance capacity) test—a reliable test for antioxidant power—kale scores a whopping 1,770, the highest in the vegetable kingdom (next best is spinach at 1,260). That means the powerful antioxidants in kale work together like the Los Angeles Lakers, bringing you the maximum firepower against cellular damage inflicted by rogue oxygen molecules known as free radicals.

Kale is also high in sulfur and contains a miraculous plant compound called sulforaphane, which boosts the body's detoxifying enzymes and may also help fight cancer in the bargain. Sulforaphane is formed when the vegetables containing it are chopped or chewed, and it triggers the liver to remove free radicals and other chemicals that may cause DNA damage. Kale is also loaded with calcium, iron, vitamins A and C, and bone-building vitamin K. It contains seven times the beta-carotene of broccoli and ten times as much lutein and zeaxanthin, vision-friendly carotenoids known to help protect against macular degeneration (the major cause of blindness in adults over 65). Plus 2 cups (40 g) of it gives you about 4 g of protein and 3 more g of fiber to add to what you are already getting from the lentils.

The other featured side here, **Steam-Baked Vidalia Onions**, of course provides lots of delicious onions. These cancer-fighting alliums contain powerful antioxidants and anti-inflammatories in addition to a whole pharmacy of nutritional compounds. You'll read all about the tremendous benefits of onions throughout this book, especially in Chapter 9.

Meal Prep Tips

- Make the Curried Quinoa Greens with Coconut Dressing ahead. It can be eaten warm or chilled.

- Use one 32-ounce (1-L) carton of broth between both the Delicious Dal and Curried Quinoa Greens with Coconut Dressing.

- Prepare the fruit for the dessert and set aside in covered bowls or store in the fridge.

- Put the Steam-Baked Vidalia Onions on to bake and then begin preparing your Delicious Dal.

- After the main meal has been eaten, prepare the fondue just before serving.

LIFE ON THE D-LIST

There's always reason to wax poetic about the health benefits of cacao, delicious in the **Raw Chocolate Fondue**. (You didn't think I was going to forget that amazing dessert, did you?) But the rest of the ingredients in the dessert aren't exactly D-list celebrities.

Strawberries contain chemicals found to protect cells against both cervical and breast cancer. They also contain ellagic acid, which has anticarcinogenic and antimutagenic activity, so much so that the American Cancer Society considers ellagic acid a very promising natural supplement. Compounds in strawberries also protect your brain and memory.

Kiwifruit was found in a study at Rutgers University in New Jersey to provide the most nutrition on an ounce-to-ounce basis of any of the twenty-seven fruits that researchers tested. It also had the highest level of vitamin C (almost twice that of an orange). And in other research, kiwis have shown the ability to protect against oxidative damage to DNA. And mangoes—well, they're just delicious. Plus they're a rich source of enzymes and they contain potassium, vitamin A, and fiber in the bargain.

Enjoy!

Low-Fat Cooking versus Healthy Cooking

I'm not a big fan of the low-fat movement. I don't think eliminating or reducing fat has a thing to do with health. On the other hand, reducing the wrong kinds of fats—and the wrong kinds of carbohydrates—has everything to do with health.

By the wrong kinds of fats I don't necessarily mean saturated fat, some of which we need. We just don't want the kind that comes from fried food. Nor do we want to eat the fat—saturated or otherwise—from animals that have been raised on factories and given antibiotics, steroids and hormones, all of which gets stored in their fat and passed on to you. But we needn't be afraid of some fat—even saturated—from grass-fed meat, wild fish, and wild game, or anything that's raised on a family farm without being fed a chemistry set's worth of carcinogens.

I'm far more concerned about two really bad sources of fat—man-made trans fats and fats that have been damaged by frying, especially in vegetable oil, which creates even more damaging compounds when it's used for deep frying than the lard it substitutes for. The biochemistry of all this is far too complicated to go into here, but the bottom line is that there's a big difference between knocking the fat out of a meal and eating healthy. High intakes of processed carbohydrates and sugar are as damaging or more damaging than fat ever was.

So here's my personal definition of healthy meals. First, healthy meals are made with whole foods, which are foods your grandmother would have recognized as food, food without bar codes. Second, healthy meals are low in sugar. Third, healthy meals are high in plant foods, but they can also be high in animal foods; both are healthy. Fourth, if possible, some ingredients should be raw. And fifth, healthy meals should be prepared lovingly and caringly with as few artificial ingredients and chemicals as possible. Finally, for overall health on a long-term basis, most healthy meals should be lower in calories than most of us are used to.

In case you didn't notice, none of that has anything to do with being low fat. But it has everything to do with being healthy.

Delicious Dal
Glucose control in every bite

Prep Time: 10 minutes
Cook Time: 35 minutes

Ingredients

2 tablespoons (28 ml) extra virgin olive oil

1 medium onion, finely chopped

3 tablespoons (24 g) fresh ginger, peeled and finely grated

4 to 5 cloves garlic, finely chopped, divided

3 cups (705 ml) water or vegetable or no-sodium-added chicken broth

1 cup (225 g) dried red lentils (may be orange, red, or salmon color), any small stones removed, well rinsed, and drained

1 teaspoon ground turmeric

2 teaspoons (10 g) ghee (clarified butter)

1 teaspoon cumin seed or ground cumin

½ to 1 teaspoon cayenne pepper

¾ cup (12 g) fresh cilantro, washed, stemmed, and coarsely chopped

3 plum tomatoes, seeded and diced

Salt

In a heavy soup pot over medium heat, heat the oil. Add the onion and sauté for about 5 minutes. Add the ginger and half of the garlic and continue sautéing over medium heat until tender, 1 to 2 more minutes. Gently pour in the water or broth, lentils, and turmeric, stirring well to combine. Increase the heat to high and cook until the mixture comes to a boil. Reduce the heat and simmer, stirring occasionally, until the lentils are tender, about 15 minutes.

While the lentils are cooking, heat the ghee in a small sauté pan over medium heat until melted. Add the cumin seed and cayenne pepper and sauté, stirring frequently, about 2 minutes, or until the cumin seed stops sizzling. Add the remaining garlic and cook another 2 to 3 minutes until very fragrant. Remove from heat.

When the lentils in the soup mixture are tender, mix or whisk the mixture well until it has a thick, creamy consistency. If you wish, you may use a soup wand to lightly purée. When the soup is pureed, stir in the ghee/spice mixture until thoroughly combined. Add the tomato and salt to taste and simmer on low for another 5 to 10 minutes. Put the dal in a tureen and pile cilantro on the middle to present. Stir it in gently just before serving.

Yield: 6 servings

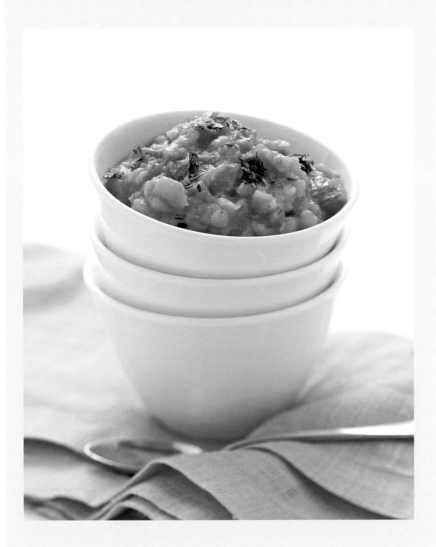

Notes from the Kitchen

- Dal (also spelled dahl) is an Indian term for a thick, souplike stew made from different varieties of legumes, usually lentils, which often includes onion and pungent spices. Nourishing and easy to digest, it is a staple in Ayurvedic cooking.

- You can serve dal alone as a starter soup or make it an entrée by serving it over simple brown basmati rice or with almond quinoa greens.

- You can buy ghee (clarified butter) at most good grocery stores. Don't look for it in the refrigerated area, though. It behaves more like cooking oil than butter, keeping well in a jar in the pantry. Simmering spices in a small amount of ghee (or butter) before adding them to a soup will bring out the richness of their flavors and punch up their aromas.

- Red-orange lentils turn golden when they cook. They are split and thus tend to turn mushy in a soup, making them a perfect choice for the consistency of a thick dal. They generally cook more quickly than brown or green lentils.

- A large, fine sieve is a helpful kitchen tool for rinsing small grains and legumes such as red lentils and quinoa.

- Simmering flavorful pungent items such as onions, garlic, or ginger in a little oil can provide a richer, sweeter flavor platform on which to build water-based soups.

- To seed plum tomatoes, cut them in half lengthwise and core them like a pepper. Then cut the remaining flesh into strips and dice into squares.

Steam-Baked Vidalia Onions

Cancer-fighter on the side

Prep Time: 5 minutes
Cook Time: 30 minutes

Ingredients

2 tablespoons (28 g) butter

3 cloves garlic, finely minced or pushed through a garlic press

2 medium Vidalia onions, peeled, ends removed, and cut in half across the middle

2 tablespoons (28 ml) water

Suggested Swaps

• Broccoli Rabe, but omit the vinegar (page 60)

• Sweet Beets and Greens, but try using red wine vinegar instead of balsamic (page 164)

Preheat the oven to 375°F (190°C, gas mark 5).

In a small sauté pan over medium heat, warm the butter until melted. Add the garlic and stir to combine and warm, about 1 minute.

Place the onions, cut side up, and the water in a small glass baking dish with a cover. Gently spoon the garlic butter onto each onion half in equal measures. Cover with the baking dish lid or an aluminum foil tent, taking care to seal edges without touching any part of the onions. Bake until the onion is soft to the fork and the garlic is lightly caramelized, about 30 minutes. Gently lift the onion out of the pan and serve.

Yield: 4 servings

Notes from the Kitchen

- These onions are an easy, low-glycemic, sweet-tasting, and sulfur-rich delight!

- When choosing onions, be aware that different types of onions have different health-promoting chemicals. The stronger-tasting ones have superior properties.

- Onion tips: Peel it under water for ease. If the onions make you cry when cutting, stick your head in the freezer for a few moments and the irritation will diminish.

- The preparation of garlic is key to its health benefits. The garlic clove has to be crushed or chopped, the more finely the better, in order for the compounds in it to interact and form allicin, which is the substance responsible for most of the good stuff garlic does.

- Allicin begins to degrade shortly after it's produced, so the fresher it is when you use it, the better. Adding chopped garlic to dishes as the last ingredient while cooking is always a good idea. Garlic experts advise crushing a little raw garlic and combining it with the cooked food shortly before serving. Allicin—the health-giving compound in garlic—is completely destroyed by microwaving. Sorry!

Curried Quinoa Greens with Coconut Dressing

Cellular damage controller

Prep Time: 10 minutes
Cook Time: 20 minutes

Ingredients

⅔ cup (120 g) quinoa

2½ cups (570 ml) water or no-sodium-added vegetable or chicken broth

3 cups (60 g) young kale, lower stems removed, and chopped into bite-size pieces

1 teaspoon curry powder

Pinch salt

3 tablespoons (45 ml) unsweetened light coconut milk

2 teaspoons (10 ml) fresh-squeezed lime juice

¼ teaspoon curry powder

¼ teaspoon agave nectar

⅓ cup (48 g) unsalted dry-roasted peanuts

In a dry, 4-quart (4-L), nonstick sauté pan over medium heat, toast the quinoa for 5 to 6 minutes until fragrant, gently turning the grains over from time to time. Add the water or broth, kale, curry powder, and salt; cover, and raise the temperature to high to bring the mixture to a boil. Lower the heat and simmer until the quinoa and kale are tender, the quinoa "tails" have popped, and the liquid is absorbed, about 15 minutes. Remove the pan from the heat and transfer the mixture to a large bowl.

In a small bowl, place the coconut milk, lime juice, curry powder, and agave nectar and whisk together briskly. Pour the coconut milk mixture over the quinoa mixture and toss to combine well. May be served warm or chilled in the refrigerator overnight. Add the peanuts just before serving.

Yield: 6 to 8 servings (about ½ cup [115 g] each)

Suggested Swaps

- Confetti Basmati Rice (page 36)
- Roasted Brussels Sprouts, Asparagus, and Broccoli with Toasted Hazelnuts, but use cashews instead of filberts (page 230)

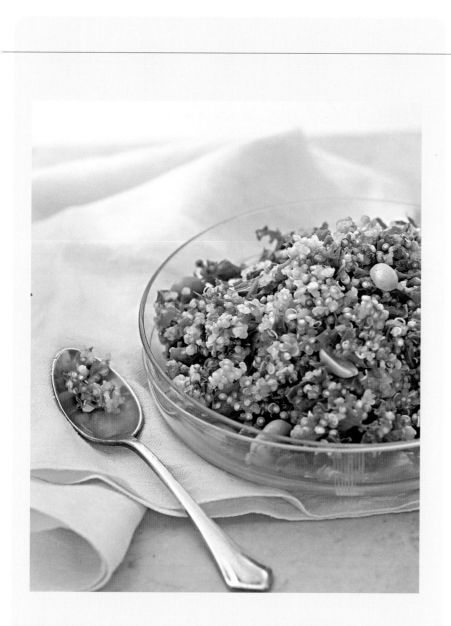

Notes from the Kitchen

- The surface of the tiny quinoa grains is coated with a bitter protective resin called saponin—a bird deterrent. To remove it before eating, either rinse the grains well under running water and drain in a fine sieve (the grains will go through most colanders) or toast lightly in a dry pan over medium heat for 3 to 5 minutes.

- Kale has a mild, cabbagelike flavor. It comes in an assortment of colors, but they all have frilly leaves. The most common types of kale in the United States have deep green leaves tinged with shades of blue or purple. Choose richly colored, relatively small bunches, avoiding limp or yellow leaves, and store them in the coldest part of the refrigerator for a maximum of three days. After three days the flavor will become distastefully strong. Remove and throw away the tough center stalk.

- If you opened a new can of coconut milk for the recipe, pour the rest into a clean ice tray and freeze into cubes overnight. Remove the cubes and store them in a freezer bag for the next time you need a small amount in a recipe. They are also great tossed into smoothies.

Raw Chocolate Fondue

Flavorful flavanols for a healthy heart

Prep Time: 10 minutes
Cook Time: None

Ingredients

1 very ripe, soft banana, peeled

¼ cup (65 g) almond butter

¼ cup (60 ml) unsweetened vanilla
almond milk

2 teaspoons (13 g) agave nectar

3 tablespoons (24 g) raw cacao or high
quality cocoa powder

½ teaspoon cinnamon, optional

½ teaspoon orange extract, optional

½ teaspoon gourmet salt, optional

½ vanilla bean (open pod and scrape
the seeds into the mix), optional

1 teaspoon Grand Marnier, optional

1 cup (110 g) fresh strawberries,
washed, stemmed, and halved

2 ripe kiwifruits, peeled and cut into
chunks or thick half-rounds

1 mango, peeled and cubed

1 cup (110 g) fresh cherries, pitted

In a blender, place the banana, almond butter, almond milk, agave nectar, and cocoa and blend well until the mixture forms a smooth cream. You can serve it as is or add any one of the following optional ingredients and lightly blend or stir in well: cinnamon, orange extract, salt, vanilla, or Grand Marnier. Scrape the fondue into an attractive serving dish. Arrange the strawberries, kiwi, mango, and cherries, or any other cubed fruit you like, in bowls with accompanying toothpicks or fondue forks for dipping and serve.

Yield: About 6 servings (makes 1 cup [230 g] of fondue)

Suggested Swaps

• Spiced Pear Sorbet (page 86)

• Grilled Pineapple (page 148)

Notes from the Kitchen

- You can use any seasonal fruit combinations. Try peaches, ripe pears, or even fresh figs for an exotic delight!

- When we think chocolate fondue, most of us think heavy cream and sugar. This delicious version has neither, but the taste remains as rich and decadent as the dish implies. Working with raw forms of all the ingredients leaves the fresh vital flavors and energy of the foods completely intact. This dessert lifts your energy rather than slowing you down. Another bonus is the ease: You need no fancy fondue warmers or other equipment, and you can have it on the table in 10 minutes flat! The primary sweetener is banana, but it broadcasts itself only slightly in the overall flavor.

- The better the cocoa you use, the better this dish will taste.

What's Up with Fiber?

Fiber—what your grandmother used to call "roughage"—is all the parts of plant food that your body can't digest or absorb. (Animal foods and fish, great as they are for their protein and fatty acids, have zero fiber.) Fiber comes in two "flavors," soluble and insoluble, and both have health benefits.

Soluble fiber, as you might expect, can dissolve in water. It forms a gel-like substance that can help lower cholesterol and blood sugar. Insoluble fiber won't dissolve, so it increases stool bulk and also moves things right along through your digestive system. Constipation can almost always be helped by adding more fiber and more water to your diet.

Soluble fiber is found in foods like apples and oats; insoluble fiber is found in the skins of fruits and vegetables as well as grains and nuts. Many foods have both.

Virtually all health organizations recommend that we get between 25 and 35 g of fiber a day in our diet. I think they're being conservative. Our Paleolithic ancestors got more than 50 g a day. The Mayo Clinic recommends 38 g for men age 50 and under. The average American gets between 8 and 11 g.

Fiber boasts an array of benefits. Check out these eight:

1. Improves blood sugar levels
2. Helps control weight
3. May reduce risk of type 2 diabetes
4. May reduce risk of irritable bowel syndrome and diverticular disease
5. Helps reduce constipation
6. Lowers cholesterol
7. Is linked to a lower risk for heart disease
8. Binds toxins and helps to eliminate them, offering protection from cancer

Note: Most commercial cereals and breads are fiber lightweights, despite what they'd like you to believe. Two exceptions are Fiber One and All Bran (extra fiber) cereals (14 g and 13 g per half cup respectively). There are others. Read the labels. Ideally you'd like 3 or more g of fiber in a slice of bread, and at least 5 g or more per serving in cereal.

What You Need to Know about Food Safety–Part I

The healthiest meals on earth can't be healthy if the ingredients in them aren't safe. Sanford Miller, Ph.D., a senior fellow at the University of Maryland Center for Food, Agriculture and Nutrition tells us to be cautious when reading labels. "Sell-by dates and 'best-used-by' labels are really about taste and appearance," he told me. "And they are always in excess of the time before it really gets spoiled. Just because a container of milk is over its sell-by date by a day or two doesn't mean it's bad." Because milk is pasteurized, pathogens are not a danger; the worst that will happen is that the milk will be sour.

Meat and poultry are a different story. All meat and poultry contain some bacteria, the most famous being salmonella and *E. coli*. "These are part of the 'natural flora' of bacteria living in all animals, including humans," Miller explained. These bacteria multiply at room temperature (or warmer) but are killed when cooked to proper temperature.

Most common bacteria don't grow at all in the cold. One less common one–listeria monocytogenes–will grow in the cold, but very slowly. "That's why it's very important that meat and poultry be kept refrigerated at all times," Miller said. Meat and poultry are safe in the refrigerator for about a week, he said.

The biggest danger with bacteria in meat and poultry comes from defrosting it on the kitchen counter, he said. "If you leave it out to defrost and forget about it, you're creating a perfect environment for the bacteria to grow in," he told me. Best advice: Always defrost in the refrigerator. Or, if you like, defrost it in the microwave, Miller advises.

Once cooked, the danger from bacteria that resided in the meat is gone, but there is always the problem of re-contamination, particularly if you leave the cooked meat out on the counter. Even cooked meat should remain refrigerated. But when meat turns grayish after a day or two, it doesn't mean anything at all. "It's the hemoglobin turning into a compound called methemoglobin, and is a normal result of being exposed to light," Miller explained.

For additional food safety tips, turn to p. 132 in Chapter 5.

Chapter 4 **Pantry List**

FOOD GROUP	FOOD
Dairy	Butter Ghee
Herbs/Spices/ Condiments	Cayenne pepper Cilantro (fresh) Cinnamon Cumin (seed or ground) Curry Powder Garlic Ginger (fresh) Gourmet salt (optional) Orange extract Salt Turmeric Vanilla beans
Miscellaneous	Agave nectar Broth (chicken or vegetable) Cacao or cocoa powder Coconut milk (unsweetened) Grand Marnier Olive oil (extra virgin) Red lentils (dried)
Nuts/Seeds	Almond butter Peanuts (dry-roasted and unsalted) Quinoa Vanilla almond milk, unsweetened
Produce	Bananas Cherries Kale Kiwifruits Lime juice (fresh squeezed) Mango Onion (Vidalia) Strawberries Tomatoes (plum)

Clockwise from top left:
Thai-Spiced Mango and Prawns, Tropical
Frosties, Roasted Rutabaga Chips,
Crunchy Coconut Fruit Salad

CHAPTER 5

Healthy Fats and Protein Packed

Thai-Spiced Mango and Prawns

MEAL:

124 Thai-Spiced Mango and Prawns

126 Crunchy Coconut Fruit Salad

128 Roasted Rutabaga Chips

130 Tropical Frosties

I'VE GOT a great story about coconut. It will probably tell you more about why you should take the nutrition info you read in magazines with a tablespoon or two of salt; but be patient, and I'll also get to the good parts about coconut.

First the story.

Not too long ago I was asked to write a story called "Healthy Foods That People Aren't Eating" for a very famous magazine. An easy assignment: I listed all the foods that people fear (such as egg yolks) and some of the many healthy foods that most people are deeply misinformed about.

And at the top of my list was coconut and coconut oil.

Fast-forward a couple of weeks. The story came back from the editor for a final fact-check and sign off. But the entire section on coconut was missing.

I called up the editorial assistant. "What gives?" I asked. The editorial assistant explained that the editor had simply taken out the section on coconut. "She doesn't think it's healthy," she said. "It has saturated fat." My jaw dropped to the floor, and I took my name off the story.

THE UNSUNG COCONUT

The prejudices against certain foods run very deep indeed. (Don't get me started on my friends who still order egg white omelets because they're afraid of the cholesterol in egg yolks.) And the reputation of coconut—so delicious here in the **Crunchy Coconut Fruit Salad**—has certainly not been helped by the American fat phobia. For far too long, this amazing, healthy, vital food has been relegated to the category of "foods that are bad for you" and forgotten about.

It's time to fix that.

The fat in coconut is largely saturated, it's true, but it's a type of saturated fat called medium-chain triglycerides, MCTs for short. These wonderful fats have some very specific qualities that make them special. For one thing, they're easy to metabolize. The body actually likes to use them for energy rather than for storage, so they're much less likely to wind up on your hips. Bodybuilders have long loved MCTs because they give them energy while dieting and are highly unlikely to put on fat.

Another quality of MCTs is that they contain a special fatty acid called lauric acid, which is a great boon to your immune system. It's antiviral and antimicrobial, has some positive effects on immunity, and according to the *Physicians' Desk Reference*, may actually be helpful against some cancers.

Fifty percent of the fat in coconut is made up of lauric acid. In the body, lauric acid forms into a compound called monolaurin, which is basically a bug killer. According to naturopath Bruce Fife, N.D., lauric acid has been shown to be effective against Streptococcus (throat infections, pneumonia, sinusitis), Staphylococcus (food poisoning, urinary tract infections), *H. pylori* (stomach ulcers), and other bacterial pathogens.

Another 6 or 7 percent of the fatty acids in coconut are an MCT called capric acid, which forms into monocaprin, a compound that has been shown to have antiviral effects and antibacterial effects against sexually transmitted bacteria. The MCTs in coconut also kill *Candida albicans* (yeast) and other fungi in the intestinal tract, further supporting healthy gut ecology.

Back in the '60s and '70s, research was done on the native diet of people from the Pacific Islands and Asia who were surprisingly free from cardiovascular disease and cancer. One study examined the diet of people living in the small, idyllic islands of Tokelau and Pukapuka. These folks ate a high-fat diet—deriving 35 to 60 percent of their calories from fat—and most of it was from coconut. Yet the islanders were blissfully free of arthrosclerosis, heart disease, and colon cancer; digestive problems were rare; and the islanders were lean and healthy. The question of the healthfulness of coconut and coconut oil should have been settled back then, but prejudices and misinformation die hard. Not to worry. There's plenty of coconut in this Thai-flavored meal to feed your immune system and support your heart.

Go a Little Coco-Nuts

When buying coconut oil, go for the best: virgin or extra virgin coconut oil. It's never hydrogenated or partially hydrogenated—meaning it doesn't contain any dangerous trans fats—and it's processed without high heat or chemicals, so you get all the nutrition that's available.

My personal favorite is Barlean's Extra-Virgin 100% Organic Coconut Oil, which comes in a tub and is widely available in stores. You can also buy it under "Healthy Foods" on my website, www.jonnybowden.com.

Try using extra virgin coconut oil as a cooking oil for eggs. Use it in place of butter or mix it with a little organic butter. Simply heat it up and fry or scramble the eggs. I start with a bunch of vegetables, let them soften for a couple of minutes, add the eggs, and mix it up. Season it with curry and lemon pepper. It's amazing. My favorite breakfast dish is to start off with some sliced apples, add the vegetables when the apple slices are transparent, and carry on with the eggs.

PROTEIN-PACKED PRAWNS

The main dish, **Thai-Spiced Mango and Prawns**, features prawns or shrimp cooked in—what else—coconut oil! Shrimp are a great source of protein, containing a whopping 17 g in a small 3-ounce serving. They're also really low in calories and loaded with a powerful antioxidant called astaxanthin, which is a member of the carotenoid family that includes better-known beta-carotene and lutein. But astaxanthin has even more antioxidant power than either of them. Some studies suggest that it can be 100 times more effective as an antioxidant than vitamin E. (Salmon, by the way, get their red color from eating the pigmented astaxanthin found in crustaceans like shrimp.)

Oh, and if you're wondering what the difference between shrimp and prawns are, the answer is not a whole lot. Mainly size. Prawns are just really big shrimp, though there are some differences of opinion about the distinctions. One particularly desirable type is the black tiger prawn, which can grow to more than a foot in length.

While we're on a myth-busting roll from our discussion of coconut, let's deal with the cholesterol in shrimp, which is one reason many people avoid eating them. Put that little piece of misinformation to rest. The cholesterol in food, such as eggs and shrimp, has virtually no effect on the cholesterol in your blood. For more than 99 percent of the population, it's highly unlikely that the cholesterol in shrimp will have any meaningful effect whatsoever on your blood cholesterol. In fact, in one study published in 1996, subjects ate 300 g of shrimp a day (approximately 12 ounces!), and although their overall cholesterol went up a bit, most of it was the good cholesterol, meaning their overall cholesterol profiles actually improved! And even more important, their triglycerides dropped. So eat and enjoy.

MORE GREAT SUPERFOODS

Here are a couple of other highlights in this meal. One of them is jicama, which I'm willing to bet many people have never heard of. Neither had I, till my friend Ann Louise Gittleman, Ph.D., C.N.S., turned me on to it. It's a root vegetable that is low calorie, high fiber, crunchy, and cooling. The high fiber of jicama alone makes it worth the price of admission, but it also comes with a little bonus serving of magnesium and potassium. You'll love it in the Crunchy Coconut Fruit Salad.

Another highlight of the Crunchy Coconut Fruit Salad is grapes, about which I can't say enough good things. The skins of dark grapes are a great source of resveratrol, which is one of the most promising antiaging compounds around. Resveratrol has extended the life span of every life form tested so far—yeast cells, fruit flies, worms, and mice—and it appears to extend life in our primate relatives as well. The seeds and skins of grapes also contain flavonoids, which help protect against the effects of internal and environmental stresses. And the latest research on grape juice, which contains the same beneficial compounds as grapes themselves, shows that it can make blood less likely to clot and increase the elasticity of blood vessels.

One more highlight of this meal is my favorite French fry substitute: **Roasted Rutabaga Chips**. This is the kind of creative thinking a chef like Jeannette, who is also a mother, comes up with when she has to deal with kids wanting to eat at McDonald's every day. Rutabagas, which are basically big fat turnips, blow the socks off white potatoes as a basis for fries. They're low in carbs, high in fiber (3.5 g per cup), and loaded with potassium. And they cost you all of about 50 calories a cup. Plus, baked rutabagas taste pretty darn good. Maybe even good enough to make your kids forget the Golden Arches.

Well, almost.

THE ANTIDOTE TO THE GOLDEN ARCHES

Speaking of kids forgetting about the Golden Arches (hey, we can dream, can't we?), wait until they taste the **Tropical Frosties** for dessert. Combining the flavor of coconut (the coconut ice cubes Jeannette came up with are pure genius!) together with banana in a nondairy base sweetened with enzyme-rich raw honey is pure joy. Your kids may never ask for a "slurpy" again after they taste this one!

Enjoy!

Meal Prep Tips

- Prepare the marinade/dressing for the Thai-Spiced Mango and Prawns first and marinate the prawns for at least 30 minutes.

- Prepare and cook the Roasted Rutabaga Chips while the prawns are marinating.

- Prepare and dress the Crunchy Coconut Fruit Salad just before cooking the prawns.

- You can blend the Tropical Frosties right before the meal and serve them along with dinner to cool the fire of the dishes, or you can serve them right afterward in traditional dessert style.

Are Shellfish (and Fish) Safe?

At first it seems simple: If shellfish and fish contain mercury, don't eat them. But the truth about shellfish and fish and mercury is a bit more complicated than it seems.

Health advisories have had to walk a fine line between scaring people away from shellfish, which is probably the healthiest source of protein and omega-3 fatty acids on the planet, and trying to control exposure to mercury. One major study found that if pregnant women were to simply replace fish high in mercury with fish low in mercury, cognitive benefits per newborn baby (of about a tenth of an IQ point) could be achieved with no loss of nutrition. But if people were scared off fish and stopped eating it, the loss of omega-3 fats during pregnancy would cut nutritional benefit by a whopping 80 percent. And if other adults—men and nonpregnant women—were to be scared off fish and decrease it even by one-sixth, risk from coronary heart disease and stroke would increase.

The fact is, many fish are also high in selenium, a fantastic mineral that binds to mercury and helps your body excrete it. The high levels of selenium in fish are believed to be responsible for the fact that people on the Seychelle Islands eat about twelve servings of fish a week with no observable problems.

I think the compromise solution offered by the Environmental Protection Agency (EPA) for women of childbearing age, pregnant women, and nursing mothers makes sense for everyone who wants to take a conservative approach. Here's what they recommend:

- Eat up to two fish meals a week of most fish, including salmon, catfish, and canned light tuna.
- Eat no swordfish, king mackerel, shark, or tilefish, which are especially high in mercury.
- Eat no more than 6 ounces (170 g) a week of albacore (white) tuna.

Personally, I think it's safe to eat fish (and shellfish) more frequently, especially if you seek out good, fresh, pure sources from reliable providers, but the EPA guidelines are a good compromise. Remember, too, that those guidelines are for those women who might become pregnant or who are pregnant or nursing. Projecting the possible risks of eating fish a few times a week for nonpregnant people is a fool's game and gets you into far more murky waters.

I'd make a major bet that any typical dinner at a fast food restaurant poses far more danger to your overall health than any fish dish I can imagine eating.

And I don't personally know any nutritionist who'd take that bet.

Thai-Spiced Mango and Prawns

Antioxidants from the sea

Prep Time: 15 minutes, marinate 30 minutes
Cook Time: 1 minute

Ingredients

5 tablespoons (75 ml) coconut milk

1 to 1½ tablespoons (15 to 22 g) Thai red curry paste

2 tablespoons (8 g) fresh cilantro, finely chopped

1 small red chili, seeds removed and finely sliced

2 cloves garlic, finely minced

Juice of 1 lime

2 ripe mangoes

2 pounds (900 g) raw tiger prawns or large shrimp, deveined and shells removed, but tails intact

2 teaspoons (10 ml) coconut oil

4 large lettuce leaves, optional

1 lime, cut into 4 wedges, optional

In a medium bowl, combine the coconut milk, curry paste, cilantro, chili, garlic, and lime juice and whisk together to blend. Set half of the mixture aside to use as a dressing on the cooked shrimp.

Peel the mangoes, then cut the side "cheeks" of flesh away and slice them into wedges. Toss the prawns or shrimp and mango wedges in the marinade and place in the refrigerator for at least 30 minutes.

Chop the remaining mango from around the stones and add it to the reserved dressing mixture.

Heat the oil in a griddle pan or wok over medium-high heat until hot. Cook the prawns and mango for approximately 30 seconds on each side, until the prawns turn pink and the mango is softened.

Arrange the prawns and mango on a serving platter or over the lettuce, if using, and drizzle with the reserved dressing. Serve with the lime, if using.

Yield: 4 servings

Notes from the Kitchen

- It takes a little while to peel shrimp, but once they are ready, the cooking time is brief. You can buy them precleaned and frozen, which is great for a quick recipe or to have on hand as an easy protein to add to a salad.

- The sweet and pungent flavors of this dish are very characteristic of Thai cooking. The cool of the fruit softens the heat of the curry paste.

- Sweet tropical fruits, such as mangoes, papayas, and bananas, are very high in sugar, so they are best eaten sparingly in season: in the high heat of summer or when you travel to hot climates.

Crunchy Coconut Fruit Salad

Feed your immune system with antiviral agents

Prep Time: 10 minutes
Cook Time: None

Ingredients

1 medium jicama, peeled and julienne cut (about 1½ cups or 195 g)

½ cup (75 g) seedless grapes, halved

2 kiwifruit, peeled and cut into thin rounds

1 large orange, peeled, one half segmented and segments cut into thirds

¼ cup (18 g) shredded unsweetened coconut

Place the jicama in a medium bowl. Place the grapes, kiwi, and orange segments on top.

In a small bowl, juice the remaining orange half (about ¼ cup or 60 ml juice) and mix with the coconut. Pour over the salad, toss well, and serve.

Yield: 4 servings

Suggested Swaps

- Citrus Avocado Salad with Nut Oil (page 38)

- Haricot Verts with Pomegranate Mint (Omit the dressing; simply serve the chilled and lightly salted beans.) (page 186)

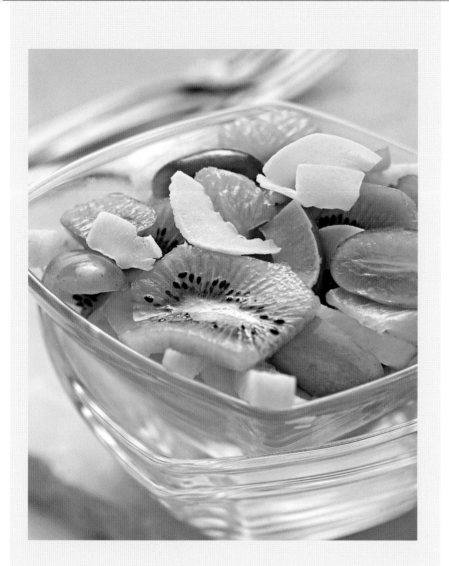

Notes from the Kitchen

- The secret sweet crunch of jicama: If you haven't yet tried this humble vegetable, now is the time to give it a whirl. It is fat-free and relatively low carb (11 g per cup with 6 g of fiber), yet it has a satisfying juicy and sweet crunch, kind of a cross between an apple and a white potato. Look for jicama with the root veggies in your supermarket. It's a tuber with a thick, tan skin. Choose a firm one with no bruising.

- Peel jicama right before using because, like an apple, it will brown slightly with air exposure.

- Jicama is great raw or lightly cooked. It stays crunchy in stir-fries.

Roasted Rutabaga Chips
Fabulously crunchy fiber

Prep Time: 10 minutes
Cook Time: 30 minutes

Ingredients

1 pound (455 g) rutabaga (1 large)

2 teaspoons (10 ml) almond oil

Cayenne pepper

Salt

Preheat the oven to 400°F (200°C, gas mark 6).

Peel the rutabaga and slice it into thin rounds. Cut each round into quarters.

In a large bowl, toss the rutabaga with the oil and cayenne pepper and salt, to taste.

Place the rutabaga in a single layer on a large baking sheet. Bake, turning occasionally, until the rutabaga is caramelized and soft, being careful not to burn, for 25 to 30 minutes.

Yield: 4 servings

Suggested Swaps

Because the Thai-Spiced Mango and Prawns has so much fruit, it's best to pair it with a simple vegetable or grain.

• Plain Brown Rice (page 292)

• Steam-Baked Vidalia Onions (Omit garlic if you wish.) (page 104)

Notes from the Kitchen

- You can use this basic recipe for many other root vegetables. It's especially good with sweet potato, parsnip, and carrots.

- Rutabagas look similar to turnips. However, turnips are smaller, thinner, and usually have white skin and tender greens. Baby spring turnips are so mild you can eat them raw as a salad radish. Rutabagas are larger than turnips and have yellow, slightly drier flesh and tougher skin. They are thought to be a cross between turnips and cabbages.

- If you do a lot of vegetable slicing, it may be worth your while to purchase a mandoline—a hand-operated utensil that can be fitted with various blades for cutting uniform slices or julienne strips. It's very helpful for slicing firmer roots and vegetables, such as rutabagas and carrots.

- While it may be unusual, we use almond oil for three reasons: First, it's a way to get the mandatory nuts in; second, it's good at high heat; and third, it has a mild flavor that complements many foods very well.

Tropical Frosties

Healthy, exotic, and enzyme-rich

Prep Time: 3 minutes
Cook Time: None

Ingredients

16 ounces (2 cups, 475 ml) chilled
    unsweetened vanilla almond milk
    (see "Notes from the Kitchen")

1½ frozen bananas (see "Notes from
    the Kitchen")

3 light coconut milk "ice cubes"
    (see "Notes from the Kitchen")

1 teaspoon raw honey, optional

Spring water ice cubes, optional

Sprinkle nutmeg, cardamom,
    cinnamon, dried coconut, or mint,
    optional

Place the vanilla almond milk, bananas, coconut milk "ice cubes," and honey, if using, into a blender and mix until smooth and creamy. Add the spring water ice cubes to taste for more thickness, if using.

If you have the bananas and coconut milk but they aren't pre-frozen, add 3 to 5 spring water ice cubes to the ingredients and blend as directed.

Divide into 4 chilled short glasses, sprinkle with the desired seasoning, and serve immediately.

Yield: 4 servings

Suggested Swaps

- Strawberry Soup (page 40)
- Real-Food Brownies (page 62)

Notes from the Kitchen

- Unsweetened almond milks are readily available in health food stores, but it is actually quite easy and much cheaper to make your own fresh: Combine 1 cup (150 g) raw almonds with 4 cups (946 ml) water in bowl. Cover and refrigerate overnight. In the morning, blend the mixture well and strain the liquid through cheesecloth, pressing it firmly to release all the milk. Store the almond milk covered in the refrigerator for a couple of days. Shake before using, because it tends to separate.

- You can substitute any milk for the almond milk. Raw cow or unsweetened rice work equally well.

- When bananas are getting overripe, freeze them for future use in frosties or smoothies. To freeze bananas, peel them, break them in half, wrap them individually in waxed paper, place them in a freezer resealable plastic bag, and freeze for at least 4 hours and up to a month.

- To make coconut milk "ice cubes," pour a can of light coconut milk into an ice-cube tray and freeze it overnight. Transfer the frozen cubes to a resealable plastic freezer bag and store them in the freezer until needed.

- For a delicious chocolate version, add 1 heaping tablespoon (9 g) raw cacao (or 2 teaspoons/6 g high-quality cocoa powder) and 1 tablespoon (20 g) agave nectar. Sprinkle with cinnamon.

- Here's another delicious and beautifully simple alternative: Peel and seed a medium-sized ripe cantaloupe or 6 cups (930 g) watermelon, chill it well (or freeze it and thin slightly with almond milk if necessary), and blend it into a creamy drink in the blender. It's light, sweet, and very refreshing!

What You Need to Know about Food Safety, Part II

Most vegetable contamination, including the recent spinach scare, comes, surprisingly, not from pesticides but from water.

"Runoffs from streams and rivers overflow the banks and get into the fields where the crops are growing," says Sanford Miller, Ph.D. "Sometimes the [food] producers even use water from these sources, and if they have been contaminated—say by animals—the crops become contaminated, too."

In the case of the spinach scare, the contamination was traced to nearby streams. While buying organic protects you from pesticides, it doesn't protect you from water contamination. "But organic farmers do tend to be more conscientious," he added.

Though there's not much the consumer can do when there's been wholesale contamination of a crop by water, the rule of thumb remains: refrigerate, refrigerate, refrigerate. "Refrigeration always slows the growth of bugs, even when something has been contaminated," Miller said.

As for fish, the best test for contamination is the smell test. "Fish should never smell fishy," Miller said. "It should smell fresh. If you even think something smells funny, throw it out. Smell is the best indicator we have that something's wrong."

Here are some highlights from the U.S. Department of Agriculture's recommendations for food safety:

- Always refrigerate food within two hours of buying (one hour when it's hot outside)
- Refrigerators should be at 40ºF (4ºC) and freezers at 0ºF (-18ºC)
- Cook or freeze meat, poultry, or fish within two days of purchase
- Wrap animal products securely and don't let meat juices get on other foods
- Wash hands with warm water and soap before and after food handling
- Cook beef, veal, lamb, roasts, and chops to 145ºF (63ºC), pork and ground meat to 160ºF (71ºC), and poultry to 165ºF (74ºC)

Get the complete set of food safety guidelines at www.fsis.usda.gov/Fact_Sheets/Basics_for_Handling_Food_Safely/index.asp

Chapter 5 **Pantry List**

FOOD GROUP	FOOD
Herbs/Spices/Condiments	Cardamon (optional) Cayenne pepper Cilantro (fresh) Cinnamon (optional) Garlic Honey (raw) Nutmeg (optional) Mint (optional) Salt Thai red curry paste
Miscellaneous	Coconut milk Coconut oil
Nuts/Seeds	Almond oil Vanilla almond milk
Produce	Banana Coconut (dried, optional) Coconut (shredded) Grapes (seedless) Jicama Kiwifruit Lettuce Lime Mangoes Orange Red Chili Rutabaga
Seafood	Raw tiger prawns (or large shrimp)

Clockwise from top left:
Spinach Soup, Striped Bass with Sun-Dried Tomato and Kalamata Paste, Grilled Pineapple, Roasted Red Pepper Dip and Crudités

CHAPTER 6

Antioxidants from the Aegean

Striped Bass with Sun-Dried Tomato and Kalamata Paste

MEAL:

142 Striped Bass with Sun-Dried Tomato and Kalamata Paste

144 Spinach Soup

146 Roasted Red Pepper Dip and Crudités

148 Grilled Pineapple

AVOCADOS were one of my favorite foods before May 17, 2007.

After May 17, 2007, they were still one of my favorite foods, but now I have an additional reason to love them. You will, too.

AVOCADOS: BURSTING WITH GOOD FATS

First some background. Avocados, which you'll love in the Spinach Soup, are one of those foods that fat-phobics tend to avoid because, well, they're believed to be "fattening." Are they? Depends. No food by itself is "fattening," but some foods are pretty high in calories. Avocados certainly are, though French fries and cheesecake both leave avocados in the dust in the calorie sweepstakes. Avocados do contain plenty of fat, but it's exactly the kind you want in your diet.

Avocados have something in common with two other great ingredients in this meal: olives and olive oil. Most of the fat in avocados and olives (and their oils) is monounsaturated fat, specifically something called oleic acid. Oleic acid, which is also known as an omega-9 fat, is one of the key features of the Mediterranean diet that's heavy on fish, vegetables, nuts, and olive oil and found in study after study to be associated with lower rates of heart disease.

Monounsaturated fat actually lowers cholesterol. In one study, forty-five volunteers who ate avocados every day for a week experienced an average 7 percent drop in total blood cholesterol. (Take that, you fat-haters!) And even more important than that drop in overall cholesterol, the ratio of good to bad cholesterol changed significantly for the better, and their triglycerides—an even more telling blood measure and an independent risk factor for coronary artery disease—dropped like a bucket. Avocados are also high in a plant compound called beta-sitosterol, which is highly protective to the prostate.

There's more good news on avocado and olive oil fat. It's been linked to a reduced risk of cancer and diabetes. And California avocados in particular happen to be loaded with lutein, a valuable member of the carotenoid family that is a natural antioxidant. It also helps your eyes stay healthy while maintaining the health of your skin.

And all that was true before May 17, 2007. Still is.

Then on May 17, 2007, researchers from Ohio State University published research that found that phytochemicals—plant compounds—in avocado were able to kill some cancer cells and prevent precancerous cells from developing into actual cancers. The lead author, Steven D'Ambrosio, Ph.D., said that avocado should be added to a list of fruits as part of a "cancer prevention diet." Specifically, the phytochemicals in avocado were effective against oral cancer, a disease with a higher proportion of deaths per number of cases than skin, cervical, or breast cancer.

So now you have yet another reason to love this amazing fruit. (Yes, trivia buffs, avocado is a fruit, not a vegetable.) And that's to add to the fact that it just tastes so darn good. In fact, the side dish of spinach, prepared with garlic, avocado, olive oil, and hazelnuts is one of the most delicious spinach dishes I've ever eaten (and that includes the legendary fried spinach dish at China Grill in South Beach, Miami!).

Florida Avocados versus California Avocados

Ah, what a difference a coastline makes! Although both varieties of avocado are absolutely wonderful for you, there are slight differences. A California avocado has about 20 percent fewer calories, about 13 percent less fat, and 60 percent fewer carbs. They're also the only one of the two that is a significant source of the two new superstars of eye nutrition: lutein and zeaxanthin. These two members of the carotenoid family support eye health and help fight macular degeneration, which is the leading cause of blindness for people over the age of 65. On the other hand, Florida avocados have about 20 percent more potassium. The bottom line: You can't go wrong with either variety.

Great Herbs and Spices for Fish

Add some zest to your fish with these spices!

Coriander seeds: If you buy them whole, crush them either with a mortar and pestle or in a designated coffee grinder to release their flavor.

Dill: If you're cooking a whole fish, place a small handful of fresh dill along with a little bit of butter into the body cavity. Sprinkle on some salt and pepper for a very tasty dish.

Marjoram and oregano: These are basically interchangeable herbs: Oregano is simply wild marjoram. Their flavor is nearly identical (aromatic and slightly bitter), with marjoram having a faint basil taste to it. Choose Turkish oregano over Mexican when cooking fish because the strong flavor of Mexican oregano overpowers fish.

Lemongrass: This herb adds a citrus touch. When using the fresh herb, it's best to throw out the outer couple of layers and then finely chop the inner leaves.

Sage: Sage should be tried with grilled tuna or other oily fish. It's best to use fresh sage because it's far less bitter than the dried version. Sage stands up well to long cooking times, making it a great choice for braised or stewed dishes.

Basil: This herb has a strong aroma, a cross between licorice and cloves. It has many different varieties. Thai lemon basil has a beautiful lime flavor that goes particularly well with fish.

A VARIETY OF VEGETABLES

It's probably not necessary to sing the praises of spinach, the headliner in this meal's **Spinach Soup**, but I will anyway. Calorie for calorie, green leafy veggies such as spinach provide more nutrients than almost any food on the planet. Spinach is a really great source of a lesser-known vitamin that happens to be critically important for building strong bones: vitamin K. This unsung vitamin activates a compound called osteocalcin that acts as a kind of glue, anchoring calcium molecules inside the bone where you want them to be. And researchers have identified no fewer than thirteen different compounds in spinach from the class of plant chemicals called flavonoids that function both as antioxidants and as anticancer agents. Spinach truly is one great food. And the soup has the added advantage of providing a really complex, robust flavor that pairs brilliantly with the beautiful crunchy raw veggies.

Of course just about everyone knows about the benefits of vegetables, but eaten raw, as they are in the **Roasted Red Pepper Dip and Crudités**, they offer an extra bonus. Raw food is loaded with live enzymes, which help you digest food and also may contribute to overall health in many ways not fully understood. Enzymes are probably the secret to why all those raw-food people look so healthy. But you don't have to become a raw-food person to get all the benefits of enzymes. Just try to get some portion of your daily diet from food that came right out of the ground or off the tree. This raw veggie salad should fill the bill nicely.

MORE THAN A FISHERMAN'S TALE

If all you know about bass is from the Sunday morning fishing shows you accidentally pass through while surfing with the remote control, it's time to dig a little deeper. Sure, bass is the mainstay of fishermen's tales, but it also happens to be a really great fish that is a healthy dietary staple as well as being the feature ingredient in this meal's main course: **Striped Bass with Sun-Dried Tomato and Kalamata Paste**. Bass is a firm, hearty fish that stands up well to grilling and strong complementary flavors. It's a great source of low-calorie protein, and one fillet has almost as much potassium as a medium-size banana.

PINEAPPLE KICKED UP A NOTCH

Speaking of enzymes, pineapple is one of the best sources of bromelain, which is a rich enzyme that helps in aiding digestion, speeding wound healing, and reducing inflammation. This delicious fruit is center stage in this meal's dessert, **Grilled Pineapple**. Now the bad news is that most of the bromelain is found in the inedible stem of the plant, but enough is left over in the delicious meaty part of the pineapple to give you a nice healthy boost. And pineapple is a great source of a little-known but essential trace mineral called manganese, which is needed for healthy skin, bone, and cartilage formation. Plus 1 cup (155 g) of pineapple gives you 2 g of fiber. And even though pineapple is sweet, its impact on your blood sugar is pretty low.

In a fit of creative flourish, Jeannette has seasoned pineapple with cayenne pepper, which is a great spice known for its metabolism-boosting effect. Hot peppers such as cayenne also contain an active ingredient called capsaicin, which is a vasodilator that enhances circulation and increases body temperature. (That's why you sometimes sweat when you bite into a hot pepper.) Cayenne pepper is used traditionally to aid digestion and stimulate the appetite; my friend Elson Haas, M.D., uses cayenne pepper as a key ingredient in his famous detox drink, the "Master Cleanser."

Meal Prep Tips

- The dishes in this meal contain a lot of complex flavors. It is best served in distinct stages.

- You'll need 45 minutes to roast the garlic, which will be used in both the Roasted Red Pepper Dip and the Spinach Soup, so that should be done in advance. If you wish to use fresh roasted peppers instead of a jarred version in the dip, roast them ahead as well.

- Make the Roasted Red Pepper Dip first and let it rest at room temperature. It is best served with crudités and a nice wine 30 minutes before the fish and soup courses.

- The Spinach Soup can sit covered at room temperature for up to five hours safely, so that can also be prepared early if you wish.

- Prepare the paste for the Striped Bass with Sun-Dried Tomato and Kalamata Paste and take the fish out of the fridge 30 minutes early if grilling.

- Prepare the pineapple for the Grilled Pineapple so it can go right onto the grill after the fish. Scrape the grill clean after the fish is complete and then grill the pineapple. Once removed, the pineapple can sit on a platter until about 30 minutes after you've finished the fish and soup course. The pineapple should be very sweet and just warmer than room temperature.

Striped Bass with Sun-Dried Tomato and Kalamata Paste

A heart-healthy Mediterranean meal

Prep Time: 5 to 10 minutes
Cook Time: 20 minutes

Ingredients

⅓ cup (18 g) sun-dried tomatoes, soaked in hot water for 15 minutes, drained, and blotted dry or if in oil, removed and drained well

¼ cup (25 g) pitted kalamata olives

2 tablespoons (28 ml) extra virgin olive oil

¼ cup (10 g) fresh basil, rinsed and dried, optional

¼ teaspoon fresh ground black pepper

2 teaspoons (6 g) capers

1½ pounds (680 g) skinless striped bass fillet

Heat grill to medium-low.

In a food processor or blender, combine the tomatoes, olives, oil, basil, and pepper. Process until the mixture forms a thick paste. Stir in the capers and set aside.

Rinse the bass and pat dry. Paint the underside lightly with olive oil and place it oiled side down on grill. After about 7 minutes, flip the bass and coat the grilled side to taste with the paste. (You will have some paste remaining. [See "Notes From the Kitchen," page 143.] Be careful not to contaminate it by touching it with any utensil that touches the uncooked fish.)

Close the grill and continue to cook for 5 to 10 minutes, or until the bass is cooked through. (It will be white and soft when pierced with a fork.) Carefully lift the bass off the grill and onto a serving plate.

Yield: 4 servings

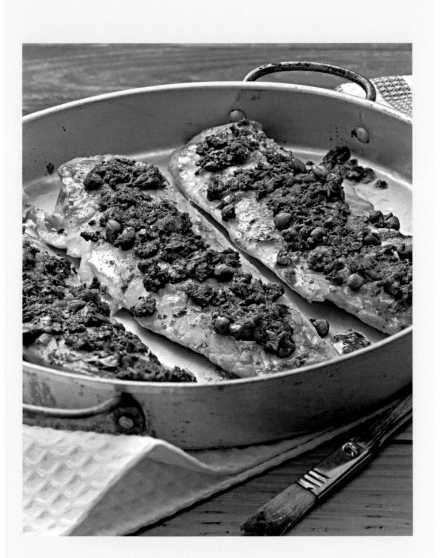

Notes from the Kitchen

- You can also bake this fish dish in the oven. Preheat the oven to 250°F (120°C, gas mark ½). Cut the bass into 4 equal pieces. Lightly oil the bottoms and place them oiled side down in a glass baking dish. Coat the top of the bass with the paste. Bake for 15 to 20 minutes, until the bass is white and soft when pieced with a fork.

- The remaining paste will keep in the refrigerator for a week and can be used like a pesto. It is wonderful with whole grain pasta or over grilled zucchini. Use it sparingly, because the flavor is very strong.

Spinach Soup

Cholesterol, cancer, and diabetes defense—all in one bowl

Prep Time: 5 to 10 minutes
Cook Time: None

Ingredients

4 cups (120 g) baby spinach, well washed and dried

1 cup (235 ml) water

2 to 3 cloves roasted garlic or 1 clove raw garlic

1-2 teaspoons (2.5-5 ml) lemon juice, freshly squeezed

Pinch salt

1 ripe avocado, cut in half and pitted

2 tablespoons (18 g) crushed dry-roasted hazelnuts, crushed raw hazelnuts, or lightly toasted pine nuts

In a blender, place the spinach, water, garlic, lemon juice, and salt. Pack the spinach leaves down and then blend until smooth, scraping down the sides as necessary.

Spoon the avocado out of its skin and into the blender and process again until smooth. Taste and add additional salt, garlic, or lemon juice if necessary. Divide into 4 equal portions and garnish with the nuts.

Yield: 4 servings

Suggested Swaps
• Confetti Basmati Rice (page 36)
• Fragrant Chard (page 204)

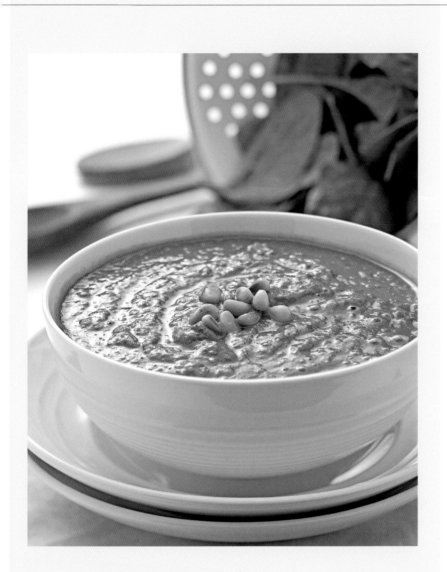

Notes from the Kitchen

- If you want to avoid cooked ingredients, omit the garlic or use raw garlic instead and use raw hazelnuts instead of dry-roasted.

- See "Notes from the Kitchen" on page 59 for some tips on cleaning spinach.

- Raw soups are very easy to make and packed with fiber and nutrients. Always use enough liquid to get the vegetable fibers to puree properly, and use avocado as a creamy base to get the proper consistency. Add the avocado last so as not to overblend. Use more or less liquid for thicker or thinner soups. You can serve raw soups at room temperature or chill them in the fridge.

- Try these recipe variations: Add a dollop of plain yogurt to each bowl in place of the nuts or omit the garlic and blend in small peeled apple for a sweeter flavor.

Roasted Red Pepper Dip and Crudités
Delicious digestive aid

Prep Time: 10 minutes
Cook Time: 45 minutes, to roast garlic

Ingredients

3 large whole bulbs garlic

1 medium red onion, peeled and sliced

1 tablespoon (15 ml) extra virgin
  olive oil

3 large roasted red peppers

2 tablespoons (8 g) fresh parsley

Dash hot pepper sauce

Fresh ground black pepper

6 cups (420 g) raw vegetable crudités,
  such as celery sticks, baby carrots,
  zucchini or summer squash spears,
  sugar snap peas, and broccoli florets

Preheat the oven to 375°F (190°C, gas mark 5).

Slice the tops off of the garlic heads so most of the cloves are exposed. Place the garlic in a pie plate or small roasting pan. Add the onion to the pan around the garlic. Drizzle the garlic and onion with the oil. Bake for about 45 minutes, until the garlic is completely soft and lightly caramelized.

Place the red peppers, parsley, garlic, onion, and hot pepper sauce in a blender and process until mostly smooth. Add black pepper to taste. Serve with the crudités.

Yield: 6 servings

Suggested Swaps

- Caesar Salad (page 294)
- Asparagus-Endive Salad (page 206)

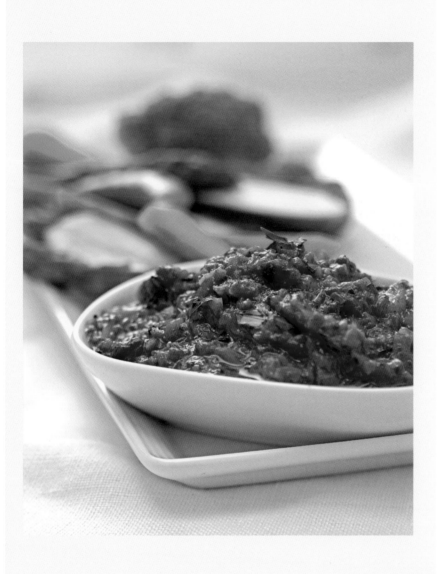

Notes from the Kitchen

- This dish has a complex, robust flavor that pairs beautifully with the sweet crunch of raw, or even steamed, veggies. It requires some roasting time to get the flavor depth, but once you have the roasted ingredients, it comes together in a flash. It's great for taking to parties.

- You can use jarred organic roasted red peppers in oil or roast them yourself. If you roast them yourself, you don't need to use any oil. Preheat the oven to 475°F (240°C, gas mark 9). Cut the peppers in half and remove the seeds and white ribbons. Place the peppers cut side down on a baking sheet. Broil the peppers for 7 to 10 minutes. Once the skins are brownish-black, remove the peppers from the oven and immediately place them in a large resealable plastic bag. Close the bag and let sit for about 30 minutes. Once the peppers are cool enough, remove them from the bag and easily peel off the skins.

- Roasted red peppers are easy to prepare anytime and will keep for a few days in the refrigerator. They are great on salads, in sandwiches, or pureed into soups.

Grilled Pineapple
A sweet treat for your skin

Prep Time: 5 minutes
Cook Time: 4 minutes

Ingredients

1 fresh pineapple, peeled, cored, and
 cut into ⅓- to ½-inch (0.8- to 1-cm)
 rings
Cayenne pepper, optional
Fresh ground black pepper, optional

Place the pineapple on a platter and sprinkle half the slices with cayenne papper, to taste, and half with black pepper, to taste. Grill each side for 2 minutes until lightly caramelized. Place gently on a plate and allow to rest until slightly cooled.

Yield: 4 to 8 servings, depending on size of pineapple

Suggested Swaps

- Real-Food Brownies (page 62)
- Silken Chocolate Parfaits (page 208)

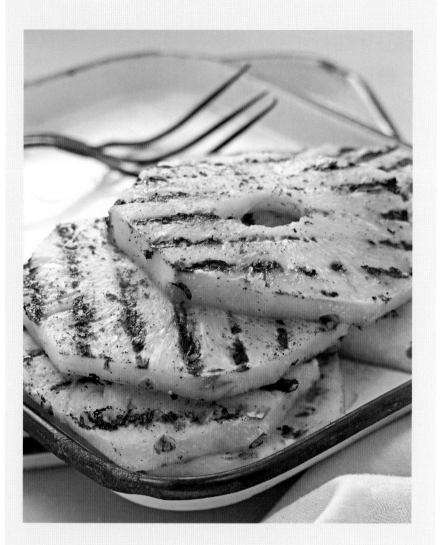

Notes from the Kitchen

- Fresh pineapple doesn't ripen after picking, so try to choose a ripe one. The leaves should be green and look fresh, and the "eyes" on the skin should be plump. The pineapple should be firm and give off a strong sweet smell of (what else?) pineapple.

- To prepare a fresh pineapple yourself, twist the crown from the pineapple, slice it in half the long way, and then quarter it. You can then cut out the core and cut off the rind. Cut the quarters into chunks. You can grill them shish-kebab style.

- To core and peel a pineapple for rings, it helps to have a proper corer and curved peeling knife, which are available at specialty stores. But most grocers sell fresh pineapple already peeled and cored for you.

- If you're concerned about the sugar content of pineapple, another tasty and quick low-glycemic hot fruit option is to halve 2 pink grapefruits, drip 1 teaspoon of raw honey onto the tops of each, and broil them in the oven for 4 to 6 minutes until lightly caramelized.

Controlling Calories with the Portion Plate

For years, we've heard that portion control is the secret to successful weight management. But we live in an era when restaurant portions have become so obscenely large that our sense of a normal size portion has become seriously distorted. Even if we were to cut those portions by one-third, we could still be eating enough to make weight loss impossible. In this context, what does portion control actually mean? And can it really work as a strategy?

Sue Pedersen, M.D., thinks it can and she's done some ingenious research to demonstrate it. Her group took 130 obese patients with type 2 diabetes and assigned them to two groups. One group received conventional care, such as standard dietary instruction (e.g., protein that would fit in the palm of your hand, a fist-sized portion of potatoes, etc). The other group received an ingenious device called the Diet Plate.

The Diet Plate is a commercially available calibrated dinner plate and breakfast bowl. The "male" version of the plate is calibrated for about 800 calories per meal, and the female version for 650. The plate is divided into four sections designed to contain pre-determined volumes of protein and carbohydrates, with small sections for cheese and sauces. The remainder of the plate is open for vegetables, which are unlimited. The cereal bowl is calibrated to allow a 200-calorie meal of cereal and half a cup of milk. The subjects were told to use the plate for the biggest meal of the day (typically dinner), and the cereal bowl for breakfast. No instructions were given regarding lunch.

"It's very hard to portion a sandwich on a plate," Pedersen told me.

The results were impressive. People using the plate were more than three times likely to lose a significant amount of weight, Pedersen said. What's more, the people using the plates were two times as likely to require a decrease of their diabetic medications.

"At the six-month mark, we even had some people who were able to come off their diabetes medications entirely," Pedersen said.

The Diet Plate used in the study is available at www.dietplate.us.

Chapter 6 **Pantry List**

FOOD GROUP	FOOD
Herbs/Spices/ Condiments	Basil (fresh) Capers Cayenne pepper Garlic Hot pepper sauce Parsley (fresh) Pepper (black, fresh ground) Salt
Miscellaneous	Olive oil (extra virgin)
Nuts/Seeds	Hazelnuts (or pine nuts)
Produce	Avocado Assorted vegetables for dipping Baby spinach Kalamata olives (pitted) Lemon Pineapple Red onion Red peppers Sun-dried tomatoes
Seafood	Skinless striped bass fillet

Clockwise from top left:
Calf's Liver and Green Onions, Sweet Beets and Greens, Sweet and Simple Almond Butter Apricot Cookies, Veggie Slaw with Flax Oil

Iron Power

Calf's Liver and Green Onions

MEAL:

162 Calf's Liver and Green Onions

164 Sweet Beets and Greens

166 Veggie Slaw with Flax Oil

168 Sweet and Simple Almond Butter Apricot Cookies

IF YOU'RE LIKE ME, you grew up when the idea of liver for dinner was about as exciting as a night spent watching *Meet the Press*. And you probably looked forward to it just as much.

Liver was—and probably still is—a tough sell. Most baby boomers remember it as the meal that tasted most like shoe leather and was supposed to be "good for you," which, at least in my house, was the kiss of death.

If that's how you remember liver, get ready to be surprised. This amazing dish is not your mother's liver, or even anything close. The thin slicing and low-temperature cooking in this recipe yields a very tender liver, and the unusual pairing of blackstrap molasses and macadamia nut oil will erase forever any childhood memory of liver and onions. Even if you are a confirmed liver hater, you should try this dish. Chances are it will win you over.

LIVER YOU'LL LOVE

First things first. There's a world of difference between beef liver and calf's liver, both for taste and for health. Calf's liver is pale pink and tender, with a subtle flavor, while beef liver is redder and tougher, with a stronger flavor. Remember that the liver is detoxification central for the body, both in humans and animals. Younger animals, such as calves, haven't been around long and therefore their livers are likely to be a lot less contaminated with the many chemicals that the cow—and every other animal on Earth—has to detoxify. This is even more so if the calf hasn't been exposed to all those chemicals in the first place, in other words if it was organically raised and grass fed. And all that means not only a healthier plate of meat, but a far more tender and tastier one as well.

Liver, which you really will love in our **Calf's Liver and Green Onions**, is a superstar when it comes to three vitamins: A, B2 (riboflavin), and B12. Vitamin A is hugely important to the immune system. Vitamin B2 is an essential nutrient that plays a key role in the production of energy.

Vitamin B12 is important for energy and metabolism, but it is very hard to get from plant foods. B12, along with vitamin B6 and folic acid, which are also in liver, make up a trio of protective nutrients that can help to reduce your level of a harmful substance called homocysteine, thereby reducing your risk of heart disease. If that isn't enough, one serving of liver has about a third of the recommended daily intake for iron.

As if you need any more reasons to try this delicious entrée, calf's liver is also cancer protective. Liver supplies about 80 percent of your recommended daily value of selenium, the best-documented anticancer mineral. Also, the riboflavin abundant in calf's liver regenerates glutathione, which is a powerful antioxidant found in every cell. It protects our cells from damage caused by free radicals, which is a long-winded way of saying it protects your cells from cancer.

Liver is also one of the best sources of protein there is. There are many different rating systems for quality of protein. I've written a few articles about those rating systems, and to tell you the truth, the details would make your eyes glaze over. The point is that there are different ways to rate the quality of protein, and no matter how you do it, liver comes out high. Nutrition Data, a website that compiles extremely detailed data on every food in the universe, uses a system they call Amino Acid Score, in which anything higher than 100 indicates a complete or high-quality protein. Liver scores 148. Enough said.

CABBAGE: A HEAD ABOVE THE REST

Besides liver, this terrific meal has an all-star list of ingredients, many of which are on the short list of superstar foods, standouts even among the greatest foods on Earth. I'm talking about cabbage, beets, apple cider vinegar, and flaxseed oil. Let's talk about each in turn.

Is It Safe to Eat Organ Meat?

Liver isn't the only organ meat. In fact, the most popular organ meats of animals are the liver, brains, and heart, while other commonly eaten foods are the stomach, kidneys, and tongue. They are powerhouses for B vitamins and excellent sources of protein. Yet a lot of people have concerns about their safety because of mad cow disease.

It's true that organ meats are all extremely perishable, so safe handling and storage are key. But beyond that, don't worry about things like mad cow disease. Humans can get a form of mad cow disease called variant Creutzfeldt-Jakob disease (vCJD) if they eat infected brain and spinal tissue, but in the past ten years only 147 cases of vCJD were reported, all in the United Kingdom except for one in the United States, and that person had been living in the United Kingdom.

Cabbage, which is front and center in **Veggie Slaw with Flax Oil**, is vegetable royalty. It's the reigning king of a brood known as the Brassica family, which includes such superstars as broccoli, kohlrabi, Brussels sprouts, and chard. For their nutritional benefits and cancer-fighting ability, cabbage—and the rest of its family—is probably the most important vegetable in the world.

The great benefits of cabbage first came to light when researchers noticed that women who lived in Eastern European countries were a lot less likely to develop breast cancer than American women. When the researchers looked closely at the differences between the diets of two populations of women, one thing that really stood out was the high intake of cabbage in the diet of Eastern Europeans. The likely compounds responsible for the lowered risk of cancer were found to be phytochemicals called indoles. Years of subsequent research have demonstrated that these indoles alter the metabolism of certain hormones in a way that is likely to reduce the risk of cancer.

But that's not all. Cabbage is also a great source of anthocyanins, which are the pigment molecules responsible for giving a vegetable or a fruit its color. (This is one reason why the darker varieties of cabbage, grapes, and the like are such nutritional powerhouses.) Those anthocyanins do a lot more than just make a plant look pretty. They also act as strong antioxidants, fighting the cellular damage done by free radicals and acting as a powerful defense against cardiovascular disease. Anti-inflammatory anthocyanins can also help dampen allergic reactions as well as help protect against the damage to connective tissue and blood vessel walls that inflammation can cause. On top of all this, cabbage is a great source of vitamins, minerals, and fiber.

Another ingredient that figures prominently in the Veggie Slaw with Flax Oil is apple cider vinegar. Much has been written touting apple cider vinegar as the uber "cure-all" for everything from weight gain to osteoporosis to arthritis. Look, let's be honest. No substance on Earth is a cure for everything. But apple cider vinegar has an awful lot of health benefits. Real unpasteurized vinegar made from apples is rich in nutrients such as potassium, and because the high heat of pasteurization kills important enzymes, real traditional unpasteurized vinegar is also a rich source of beneficial enzymes. And recent research has actually found that apple cider vinegar significantly improved insulin sensitivity in insulin-resistant subjects. If that sounds a bit technical to you, the point is simply that it helps people who have trouble managing their blood sugar manage it better. My friend Jeff Volek, Ph.D., R.D., suggests a salad with vinegar at the beginning of every meal just for its potential help with managing blood sugar.

The other "named" ingredient in Veggie Slaw with Flax Oil, flaxseeds, along with their oil, have been correctly praised for being a health food since the term health food was first invented! Flax is one of the plant kingdom's only sources of omega-3 fats, and for strict vegetarians, flaxseed oil may be their only hope of getting omega-3s in their diet. Flaxseed oil, used here in Veggie Slaw with Flax Oil, tastes great, it has anti-inflammatory properties, and—if you buy a really high-quality brand such Barlean's, which is organic, cold pressed, and made in small batches—you're also likely to get a nice dose of lignans, which are plant compounds that have a protective effect against hormone-sensitive cancers such as breast, uterine, and prostate.

BEETS? SWEET!

Another superstar vegetable in this meal that doesn't get nearly enough attention is beets. They're delicious in **Sweet Beets and Greens**. In many holistic, integrative, and Eastern traditions, beets are considered to be a super blood purifier and liver tonic. They're an important dietary source of both betaine and folate, two nutrients that play important roles in the health of the cardiovascular system by helping to break down and reduce toxic levels of an inflammatory compound in the blood called homocysteine. (High levels of homocysteine put you at seriously increased risk for Alzheimer's, heart disease, and stroke.) And beets are a really good source of potassium. Two small beets contain quite a lot more than a medium banana.

Meal Prep Tips

- Make the Sweet and Simple Almond Butter Apricot Cookies ahead. They keep well for a few days in a tightly closed container at room temperature or in the refrigerator.

- Make the Veggie Slaw with Flax Oil ahead, too, because the flavor improves with a little time for the ingredients to combine.

- Start the mealtime preparation with the Sweet Beets and Greens and cook the Calf's Liver and Green Onions while the Sweet Beets and Greens are steaming.

KEEPING IT SWEET AND SIMPLE

This meal's dessert, **Sweet and Simple Almond Butter Apricot Cookies**—which is delicious, by the way, like all of Jeannette's concoctions—is made with eggs. Eggs are one of my favorite foods to talk about, as many magazine writers who interview me can attest to. (And attest to. And attest to. If you get my drift.) I like talking about eggs because I like doing my part to rescue their reputation from the clutches of the no-fat crowd who convinced America that we need to fear eggs because of their cholesterol and fat content, which is another piece of misinformation perpetuated by the moribund American Dietetic Association. I've written about eggs at length (see *The 150 Healthiest Foods on Earth*), but let me highlight some of the important myth-busting points here.

- You don't need to fear the cholesterol in eggs. Dietary cholesterol has virtually no impact on your blood cholesterol.

- A jumbo egg has about 6 g of fat, about half of which is heart-healthy monounsaturated fat, and the other grams are nothing to worry about.

- No study has ever shown that people who eat more eggs have higher rates of heart disease or mortality than non-egg eaters.

Those are the reasons not to fear eggs. Here are the reasons to love them.

- Egg yolks are a major source of two of the most eye-healthy nutrients on the planet: lutein and zeaxanthin.

- Egg yolks contain choline, which is an important precursor of the neurotransmitter acetylcholine, which is vitally important for memory and thinking. Yup, eggs are brain food!

- Whole eggs are one of the highest-quality protein foods on the planet.

- In 2001, Kansas State University researchers identified a substance in eggs called phosphatidylcholine that blocks any LDL—or "bad"—cholesterol from entering the bloodstream.

To sum up, this is a surprisingly great meal—surprising only because most people can't believe liver can taste this good. You'll feel like you got healthier just looking at the salad and the beets. And the dessert is lovely.

Enjoy!

Artificial Sweeteners versus Natural Sweeteners

Here's the dirt on artificial sweeteners. Whether we're talking about forms of aspartame (Equal and Nutrasweet) or saccharin (Sweet 'n Low, Splenda, or sucralose), they are all chemicals, they are all toxic to the body, and they are all unhealthy.

Aspartame is made up of three chemicals that when ingested and heated up in the body become toxic substances that have been linked to some cancers and the production of neurotoxins.

Saccharin, which has been around for more than 100 years, is 300 times sweeter than sugar with a noticeable aftertaste.

Metabolically, excessive amounts of a substance called phenylalanine, found in artificially flavored foods and drinks, can also greatly affect mood by causing a decrease in the levels of the mood regulator serotonin. As a result, carbohydrate cravings go up and the thought of a successful diet goes out the window. Artificial sweeteners, therefore, can sometimes contribute to compulsive eating instead of controlling overeating. In fact, in one study at the University of Texas, the risk of obesity increased 41 percent for every can of diet soda consumed.

Banish artificial sweeteners from your diet if you possibly can. Switch to xylitol, an FDA-approved natural sweetener, which is also known as birch sugar and classified as a sugar alcohol. It does not carry any undesirable side effects, does not alter blood sugar balance (it scores a low 7 on a glycemic index scale of 100, so it's ideal for people with both diabetes and a sweet tooth), and does not sabotage your mood and energy levels. Other natural sweeteners are stevia, a south American herb, honey, and Lo Han.

There really is no reason to resort to unhealthy, risky artificial sweeteners when there are other natural, better options available. Once you make the switch, you'll have a hard time tolerating the aftertaste of the artificial, toxic substances.

Calf's Liver and Green Onions

High-quality protein, iron, and vitamins

Prep Time: 5 to 10 minutes
Cook Time: 15 to 20 minutes

Ingredients

1 pound (455 g) calf's liver, membrane removed

1 tablespoon (20 g) blackstrap molasses

⅓ cup (80 ml) no-sodium-added chicken broth

½ teaspoon salt or to taste

½ teaspoon black pepper

8 green onions (about 1 big bunch), washed, roots removed, top 3 inches (8 cm) of greens removed and chopped into ¼-inch (0.6-cm) pieces

2 tablespoons (15 g) whole wheat pastry flour (see "Notes from the Kitchen")

1 tablespoon (8 g) mustard powder

1 tablespoon (15 ml) macadamia nut oil

Using a very sharp knife, slice the liver on an angle into 4 long thin pieces no thicker than ½ inch (1 cm) each. Set aside.

In a small bowl, whisk together the molasses, broth, salt, and pepper. Stir in the onions. Set aside.

On a sheet of waxed paper or a plate, combine the flour and mustard powder. Dredge the liver pieces in the flour mixture until lightly coated.

In a large skillet, heat the oil over medium-high heat for 2 to 3 minutes, until hot. Add the liver and brown lightly for about 1 minute on each side. Pour the broth mixture over the liver.

Reduce the heat to low and cook for 15 minutes, or until the liver is cooked through but still light pink on the inside. If necessary, remove the liver to a plate, covering to keep warm, and cover the pan, softening the onions for another 2 to 4 minutes. Cover each slice of liver with equal portions of onion broth glaze and serve.

Yield: 4 servings

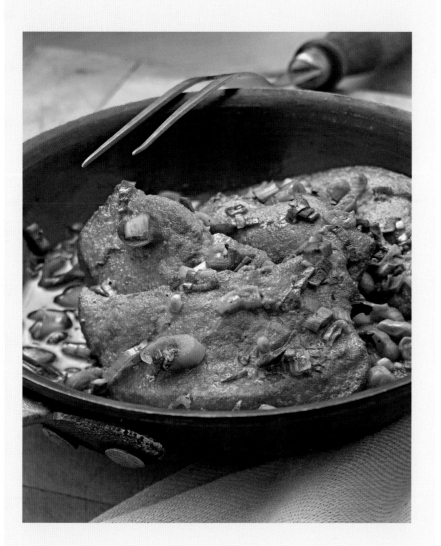

Notes from the Kitchen

- Although we generally avoid flour in our recipes, in this case the small amount of flour is helpful because it protects the meat from forming advanced glycation end-products that result from protein destruction when browning meat.

- Seek out meat producers known for humane treatment of calves. We never endorse commercial veal. See Sources for Specialty Ingredients on page 358 for some suggestions about where to get grass-fed meat and meat products from humane sources.

- Like all organ meats, liver is very perishable. Refrigerate liver at very cold temperatures for only 1 to 2 days. If you don't think that you'll cook it by then, pack it tightly and store it in the freezer for up to 4 months.

Sweet Beets and Greens

A potent potassium-strong side

Prep Time: 10 minutes
Cook Time: 40 to 50 minutes

Ingredients

6 medium whole beets (about 2 bunches), greens removed and set aside

1 tablespoon (15 ml) balsamic vinegar

3 tablespoons (45 ml) extra virgin olive oil, divided

2 tablespoons (28 ml) water

Dash salt and black pepper or freshly squeezed lemon juice, optional

2 medium shallots, finely chopped

Beet greens, well washed and coarsely chopped

Scrub the beets well and steam them whole over boiling water for about 30 minutes for small or medium beets or about 40 minutes for large beets. Then run the beets under cold water and gently peel off the skins with your fingers. Chop them into bite-size chunks and place them in a medium bowl.

In a small bowl, whisk together the vinegar, 2 tablespoons (28 ml) of the olive oil, the water, and the salt, pepper, or lemon juice, if using. Pour the mixture over the beets and set aside.

In a large sauté pan, heat the remaining tablespoon (15 ml) olive oil over medium-low heat. Add the shallots and sauté for 2 minutes. Add the chopped greens and cover. Simmer for 5 to 7 minutes, until the greens are wilted. Add the beets and heat through for a minute or so. Serve immediately.

Yield: 4 to 6 servings, depending on the beets' size

Suggested Swaps

- Fragrant Chard (page 204)

- Roasted Brussels Sprouts, Asparagus, and Broccoli with Toasted Hazelnuts (Try substituting walnuts or pecans for the hazelnuts.) (page 230)

Notes from the Kitchen

- Beets and their greens complement each other very nicely, but the greens are so perishable that it's not always easy to find them intact. Look for the freshest ones at your local farmers' market in the summer.

- If you have a pressure cooker, you can use that to save time cooking harder vegetables such as beets and turnips.

- Shallots are a lovely pungent vegetable with a rich taste similar to sweet onion with a hint of garlic. You can differentiate them from onions by their copper-colored papery skin and long, tapered shape. Shallots can make you cry when you cut them, like onions, but they generally have a milder flavor.

Veggie Slaw with Flax Oil

A cancer-fighting coleslaw

Prep Time: 20 minutes if hand-cutting, 10 minutes with food processor
Cook Time: None, but flavors improve with resting time of a couple of hours

Ingredients

2½ tablespoons (35 ml) flaxseed oil or extra virgin olive oil

2½ tablespoons (35 ml) raw apple cider vinegar

2½ tablespoons (35 ml) fresh lemon juice

¼ teaspoon sodium-free lemon pepper

½ small-to-medium head red or green cabbage, cored, quartered, and thinly sliced

3 stalks broccoli, crowns removed, peeled, and thinly sliced

4 carrots, grated or thinly sliced

4 stalks celery, thinly sliced

In a large bowl, combine the oil, vinegar, lemon juice, and lemon pepper and whisk together to combine. Add the cabbage, broccoli, carrots, and celery. Toss to coat with the dressing. Refrigerate for several hours. This will keep well for up to a week if you keep it cold and tightly sealed.

Yield: 8 to 9 cups (720-810 g)

Suggested Swaps

• Haricot Verts with Pomegranate Mint (Omit dressing and serve the salted and chilled beans.) (page 180)

• Caesar Salad (page 294)

Notes from the Kitchen

- You can use either red or green cabbage, but the red (also known as purple) makes a beautiful salad.

- The dressing is great made with Barlean's Omega Twin, which is a winning omega-3, -6, and -9 combination of flaxseed and borage oils. You can find it at most natural food stores. The longer the salad "rests," the more you'll taste its subtle flavors.

- Never cook with flaxseed oil, or any other omega-3 oil for that matter. These fats are delicate and easily damaged at cooking heat. You can pour flaxseed oil on anything, including steamed vegetables, but don't heat it in the pan!

- If you have the time, it's very meditative to chop all the veggies by hand. But you can put each of these vegetables through the food processor fitted with the slicer blade. This cuts your chopping time down to almost nothing. The easiest option of all is to buy precut versions of everything in bags; there is a great product with broccoli, cabbage, and carrots, all julienned together!

- I like Frontier brand lemon pepper, available at most natural grocers.

- To make this salad a summer meal by itself, simply throw a little cold chicken or canned tuna on top. Because the flaxseed oil has such a strong flavor, "slaw" salads with citrus, cider vinegar, and raw cabbage (all strong and complementary flavors) are a great way to add more flaxseed oil to your diet.

Sweet and Simple Almond Butter Apricot Cookies

Boosts your brainpower

Prep Time: 5 to 10 minutes
Cook Time: 12 minutes

Ingredients

1 cup (260 g) roasted almond butter
   (see "Notes from the Kitchen")

⅔ cup (16 g) xylitol

1 egg

¼ teaspoon vanilla or almond extract,
   optional

⅓ cup (43 g) dried apricots, chopped
   to pebble size (easiest in food
   processor)

Preheat the oven to 350°F (180°C, gas mark 4).

Using an electric mixer, beat the almond butter and xylitol together until well blended. Add the egg, vanilla or almond extract, and apricots and mix well. Form 1-inch (3-cm) balls and place them in rows on a large, ungreased baking sheet. With a fork, make a crisscross pattern on each cookie to flatten somewhat.

Bake for 12 to 14 minutes. (Oil will pool around the cookies as they cook.) Allow the cookies to cool thoroughly on the baking sheet to keep them from crumbling.

Yield: 25 to 30 cookies

Suggested Swaps

• Real-Food Brownies (page 62)

• Silken Chocolate Parfaits (page 208)

Notes from the Kitchen

- These cookies will keep for a few days in a tightly closed container. Store them in the refrigerator for a chewier texture.

- To reduce the fat of these cookies, simply drain the oil off the top of your jar of almond butter rather than mixing it back in.

- These dense, sweet, chewy cookies are very satisfying. They are high in fat because of the nut butter, but the fats are high quality, and they are low in carbohydrates.

- Try some easy variations of these delicious cookies. You can substitute peanut butter for the almond and omit the apricots. And for a special variation, throw in grain-sweetened dark chocolate chips.

- These gluten-free cookies are great for people with gluten allergies or celiac disease.

- Though nut butters such as the almond butter used in the dessert are enormously healthy, they're also very high in calories. So if weight loss is a goal, substitute another dessert or keep your portion really small.

Cooking with Xylitol

Here are some facts about xylitol.

- Xylitol has 40 percent fewer calories than sugar and has 2.4 calories per gram.

- Xylitol has a low glycemic index.

- It is a naturally occurring sugar that's safe for people with diabetes and hypoglycemia.

- Xylitol has a cooling effect, making it great to use in your home ice cream makers!

Getting the Most out of Snacks and Mini-Meals

You may have heard that eating frequent, small meals is the healthiest way to eat. While that's not a complete myth, neither is it the whole truth. People differ widely in their response to frequent eating, and many people actually do much better on three simple meals a day with nothing in between. But many also do better with more frequent smaller meals or a combination of meals and snacks.

That said, most people find themselves wanting a snack from time to time. Wherever you are on the continuum, following a few basic rules can make your snacks (or, as they're sometimes called, "mini-meals") part of a lifestyle based on the healthiest meals on earth. Just think of each snack—or mini-meal—as a mini version of the polymeal. It may not contain all the ingredients that a complete polymeal would, but the more the better.

The only difference between a snack, a mini-meal, and a full meal is the amount of food. Think of a snack as a toy-sized version of a meal, a mini-meal as just that—a meal in miniature—and a full meal as the grownup version. As a rule of thumb, a good snack should be 100-200 calories, a mini-meal up to 300-400 calories, and a full meal anywhere from 300-800. Our own personal preference is to try to save meals of more than 800 calories for rare occasions, like an annual feast!

Follow these three rules for the best of all possible worlds when it comes to snacks and mini-meals:

1. Quality snacks with staying power are more than just temporary fillers; look for snacks high in fiber or with some protein. A protein shake with added flaxseeds for fiber or with high-fiber berries is an example. Or try high fiber, whole grain crackers with a small amount of cheese. Nuts with a few raisins thrown in for good measure are another good choice.

2. Be prepared—keeping a regular stock of different kinds of snack foods available in your pantry, in your car, and at work will help prevent both grabbing lower quality options and overeating.

3. Quality counts. In general, fresher and less refined food contains more nutrition and long-lasting energy.

Chapter 7 **Pantry List**

FOOD GROUP	FOOD
Dairy	Eggs
Grains	Flour (whole wheat pastry)
Herbs/Spices/Condiments	Balsamic vinegar Black pepper Lemon pepper Mustard powder Salt Vanilla extract (or almond)
Meat	Calf's liver
Miscellaneous	Blackstrap molasses Broth (chicken) Olive oil (extra virgin) Raw apple cider vinegar Xylitol
Nuts/Seeds	Almond butter Flaxseed oil (or olive oil) Macadamia nut oil
Produce	Apricots (dried) Beets (whole, with greens) Broccoli Cabbage (red or green) Carrots Celery Green onions Lemon Shallots

Clockwise from top left:
Persian-Style Chicken with Walnut,
Onion, and Pomegranate Sauce;
Cauliflower "Cream"; Haricot Verts
with Pomegranate Mint; Baked Apples

CHAPTER 8

Nourishing and Nutrient-Filled

Persian-Style Chicken with Walnut, Onion, and Pomegranate Sauce

MEAL:

182 Persian-Style Chicken with Walnut, Onion, and Pomegranate Sauce

184 Cauliflower "Cream"

186 Haricot Verts with Pomegranate Mint

188 Baked Apples

CHICKEN, apples, walnuts, butter, blackstrap molasses, dried cherries, pomegranate juice, and honey. If that list of ingredients doesn't make your mouth water, I don't know what will. And every one of them can be found in this original, cleverly balanced meal of usual and not-so-usual ingredients mixed together for a veritable health bonanza.

What gives the **Persian-Style Chicken with Walnut, Onion, and Pomegranate Sauce** its unique flavor and feel is the combo of pomegranate juice and walnuts (or pecans) sweetened with iron- and mineral-rich blackstrap molasses, which is one of the best sweeteners on the planet. Read on.

AND THE OSCAR GOES TO ... POMEGRANATE

In my book *The 150 Healthiest Foods on Earth*, I wrote that if pomegranate juice were an actress, it would be considered a "rising star." Though pomegranate juice was practically unknown in the United States just a few short years ago, it has since been the subject of a ton of research, and the results have been so impressive that even mainstream medicine is paying attention to this new star on the superfood horizon. Pomegranate juice is protective against heart disease and cancer, plus it's even been called "a natural Viagra"! (I knew that would get your attention!)

Research recently published in the *Journal of Urology* examined the effect of long-term intake of pomegranate juice on erectile dysfunction. The researchers established that free radicals—those rogue molecules that can damage your cells and DNA—have a profound effect on erectile dysfunction. Enter the juice of the pomegranate. Because of pomegranate juice's powerful antioxidant capabilities, it can help quench the free radicals and do damage control on their ability to harm cells. In earlier research done in Israel and California, scientists tested a bunch of juices and other drinks for antioxidant capacity and found that pomegranate juice scored the highest of any drink they tested, including red wine and green tea. To that extent, it just might deserve the nickname "natural Viagra."

Pomegranate also has the capacity to slow aging and protect against disease. In one study, forty-eight men who had been treated for prostate cancer with either surgery or radiation were given eight ounces of pomegranate juice to drink daily. Drinking the juice significantly lengthened the time it took for the men's average PSA numbers (a marker for prostate cancer) to double. While the juice didn't stop the progression of the disease, it significantly lengthened the time it took to develop, indicating that there may be chemicals in the juice that have some cancer-fighting benefits.

Then there's the heart. In a study published in the *American Journal of the College of Cardiologists*, eight ounces of pomegranate juice were given to forty-five patients who had ischemic heart disease. Compared to non–juice drinkers, the patients drinking the pomegranate juice had less oxygen deficiency to the heart during exercise, suggesting improved blood flow to the heart. Not only that, pomegranate has shown that it has the ability to inhibit oxidation—or damage—to LDL ("bad") cholesterol. Because LDL is only a real problem in the body when it's oxidized, anything preventing oxidation is a bonanza for the heart and for cardiovascular health in general. Meanwhile, a number of other studies have shown a beneficial effect of pomegranate juice on cardiovascular health, including one that showed that it reduced arterial plaque.

The Best Salt to Use

Believe it or not, all salt is not the same. The healthiest type of salt to use is a high-quality, unrefined sea salt, not the typical iodized salt you find so nicely packaged at the grocery store. Truth be told, that all-too-common table salt, which comes from salt mines, has been dried at extremely high temperatures, altering its chemical structure and thus stripping away many of its beneficial elements. What remains in this process is sodium chloride, a substance that's actually foreign to the body (kind of like those trans fats I rant about). To top it off, harmful additives and chemicals (such as aluminum silicate) are often added in during processing.

On the other hand, unrefined sea salt, which is harvested from a living ocean or sea, contains a wonderful array of elements that the body can benefit from, including iron, magnesium, calcium, potassium, manganese, zinc, and iodine. One noticeable difference is that you won't get that typical bloating that results from using regular table salt. And for the icing on the cake: Sea salt is most definitely more flavorful than your typical table salt.

AS HEALTHY AS MOLASSES IN JANUARY

Another superstar food in this meal is blackstrap molasses. I said it's one of the best sweeteners on the planet, and here's why. Molasses is actually the by-product of sugar refining, the stuff the white sugar producers leave behind because nobody wants it. But it actually contains all the nutrients from the raw sugarcane plant. Because the roots of the sugarcane plant grow pretty deep, they're able to receive a broad range of minerals and trace elements from those deep layers of the soil. Then, when sugarcane is refined, the plants are boiled to a syrup from which the crystals are extracted. Then the plants are boiled two more times, both of which produce molasses, but blackstrap molasses only comes from the third and final boiling. It's essentially the "dregs" of the barrel, but it contains the most nutrition. It has a low amount of sugar and a high amount of nutrients, including iron, potassium, calcium, magnesium, and especially manganese and copper. And although blackstrap molasses has the least amount of sugar of the molasses family, it has more than enough to impart a delicious taste of unusual sweetness to this remarkable chicken dish.

"KING" CAULIFLOWER AND OTHER SUBJECTS

When I'm giving my general nutritional recommendations in "shorthand" at seminars, I often say something like "get the white stuff out," meaning ban anything white from your diet. But I remind people that there are a few exceptions—very few—to that rule. One of them is cauliflower, one of the few "white things" that's actually good for you.

Cauliflower, featured in this meal in **Cauliflower "Cream,"** is a member of that famous family of vegetable royalty, the Brassica family, which also includes cabbage and Brussels sprouts. Cauliflower contains indoles, a group of potent cancer fighters, and it also contains a phenomenal plant chemical called sulforaphane. Sulforaphane is a potent antioxidant and stimulator of natural detoxifying enzymes in the body.

The Cauliflower "Cream" is one of the most amazing substitutes for mashed potatoes I've ever tasted. I think it was Arthur Agatston, M.D., the South Beach Diet pioneer, who first started promoting cauliflower as a substitute for potatoes, and this recipe concept, suggested by our friend Lora Ruffner of Low-Carb Luxury fame, is always a crowd pleaser.

Haricot verts, as in the **Haricot Verts with Pomegranate Mint**, is the French term for green beans. Green beans contain folate and a bunch of other vitamins in small amounts, such as calcium, vitamin A, and potassium. They also contain about 20 percent of the Daily Value for manganese, a key trace mineral that's important for growth, reproduction, wound healing, brain function, and metabolizing sugars, insulin, and cholesterol.

AN APPLE A DAY KEEPS DISEASES AWAY

Then for dessert, there's **Baked Apples,** spiced up with butter, dried cherries (or goji berries), cinnamon, cloves, and rolled oats. Grandma was right: An apple a day really does keep the doctor away. And as it turns out, probably a whole lot more than just the doctor. When researchers examined the dietary habits of more than 34,000 women in the Iowa Women's Health Study, they found that three foods stood out for their significant ability to lower both the risk of coronary heart disease and cardiovascular disease: apples, pears, and red wine.

The reason? Plant compounds called flavonoids. Based on food-frequency questionnaires and data from the U.S. Department of Agriculture, researchers were able to approximate the flavonoid consumption of the women and calculate the impact of those flavonoids on their health. The results were impressive. Flavonoid-rich foods such as apples were associated with significant reduction in heart disease and overall mortality.

In the coloring of fruits and vegetables, there are thousands of molecules known collectively as polyphenols. Flavonoids are one particular class of these polyphenols. And the most abundant, most bioavailable, and most studied of these flavonoids is a compound called quercetin. Apples are a significant source of quercetin, which has quite a résumé of health benefits.

Meal Prep Tips

- The Cauliflower "Cream" is delicious, but it's optional. If you're trying to save time, you can omit it. But Cauliflower "Cream" makes a great alternative to mashed potatoes when you're craving warming, nourishing comfort food.

- You can make the Haricot Verts with Pomegranate Mint ahead of time and let it chill in the fridge.

- Begin the meal prep with the Baked Apples. The wonderful aroma of baking apples will permeate your whole kitchen.

- When the apples are in the oven, begin the Persian-Style Chicken with Walnut, Onion, and Pomegranate Sauce.

- Once the chicken is simmering, prepare the Cauliflower "Cream."

The quercetin in apples is, interestingly enough, in the peel, so for goodness' sake, when you bake apples never peel them. The peel prevents the harmful effects of the UV rays of the sun from hurting the fruit and also prevents microbes from getting in. So quercetin is the first line of defense for the apple. It appears to have many of these same protective effects on human cells. Quercetin impacts the immune system, reacts against cancer cells, and is a powerful anti-inflammatory. Quercetin has been linked to a reduction in heart disease as well as to a reduction in lung cancer.

The polyphenols found in fruits such as apples act as both anti-inflammatories and antioxidants. In cardiovascular disease, inflammation and oxidation very much hasten or augment the process of plaque buildup, so anything that reduces inflammation and oxidation—such as quercetin and the other flavonoids in apples—is going to help.

This most recent study is just the latest in emerging research showing that what we eat can have a profound effect on our risk for a number of degenerative diseases. While the research continues to accumulate, it makes awfully good sense to keep eating as many fruits and vegetables as possible. After all, that's where compounds like the flavonoids are found in abundance. As a nice added touch, the baked apple is peppered with goji berries, which are kind of a cross between a cranberry and a cherry. Goji berries have been used in Tibet and China for hundreds of years and are regarded as a longevity, strength-building, and sexual potency food of the highest order.

Enjoy!

Free-Range Chicken: Grand Slam or Grand Scam?

Let me be honest. I always buy free-range chickens and eggs from "cage-free" hens. I'm also increasingly suspicious of whether those terms mean anything.

In an ideal world, the chickens that we eat would run around on small family farms, pecking away at the ground to forage for their natural diet of worms and insects and all the other omega-3-rich foods they would naturally eat. They'd get exercise, so they wouldn't be so fat. They'd come from organic, conscientious farms so their bodies wouldn't be filled with the growth hormones and antibiotics that the poultry industry uses on factory-farmed animals.

But this is far from an ideal world. Chickens are among the most abused animals on the planet. They're packed by the thousands into filthy sheds, and each chicken has about as much space as a sheet of paper. They are fed massive amounts of antibiotics and drugs, including hormones to make them grow large and fast. They're typically slaughtered at seven weeks or less, years short of their normal life span.

Free range and organicare labels we hope would assure us that the animals we eat had a life different from the one I just described. Free-range animals, in principle at least, are permitted to roam freely and live in natural surroundings. But unfortunately, there are few regulations on the term free range, and you can be pretty sure that it's only a matter of time before the term becomes so diluted that it loses any real meaning. To give a "free-range" certification, the USDA simply requires that chickens have access to the outdoors. The key word is access. Often "access" simply means a little "doggy door" that few chickens even recognize, let alone use.

But yes, with all that said, I still buy free-range chickens. I like to hope that I have a better chance of getting a bird that had some semblance of a normal life, eating its normal diet, and ultimately—dare I hope—slaughtered humanely. Free-range, organic chicken—if it really is free range—is a healthier, tastier meat with less of the toxins I'd rather not have in my diet.

And buying free range lets me sleep a little better at night.

Persian-Style Chicken with Walnut, Onion, and Pomegranate Sauce

A delicious disease-fighter and anti-aging entrée

Prep Time: 5 to 10 minutes
Cook Time: 40 minutes

Ingredients

3 tablespoons (45 ml) unsalted butter or olive oil

2½- to 3-pound (1- to 1¼-kg) chicken, cut into serving pieces (see "Notes from the Kitchen")

2 medium onions, thinly sliced

1 teaspoon ground cinnamon

2 cups (220 g) toasted walnuts or pecans, coarsely ground

⅔ cup (157 ml) pomegranate juice

½ cup (123 g) tomato sauce

1½ cups (355 ml) no-sodium-added, fat-free chicken broth

1 tablespoon (15 ml) plus 1 teaspoon freshly squeezed lemon juice

¼ teaspoon salt

¼ teaspoon ground black pepper

1 tablespoon (20 g) blackstrap molasses

In a large, heavy skillet or Dutch oven, heat the butter or oil over medium-high heat until melted and the foam subsides. Sauté the chicken, turning it occasionally, for 10 to 15 minutes, or until it is browned on all sides. Transfer the chicken to a plate. Reduce the heat to medium-low and add the onion to the skillet. Sauté, scraping up brown bits, for 10 minutes, or until it is golden and softened. Stir in the cinnamon and continue to cook, stirring constantly, for 1 more minute. Stir in the walnuts or pecans and cook the mixture, stirring, for 1 more minute. Stir in the pomegranate juice, tomato sauce, broth, lemon juice, salt, pepper, and molasses. Bring the mixture to a boil and simmer for 3 minutes. Add the chicken, leaving any juices that have accumulated on the plate, reduce heat, and simmer the mixture, covered, for 15 to 20 minutes, or until the chicken is cooked through.

Yield: 4 to 6 servings

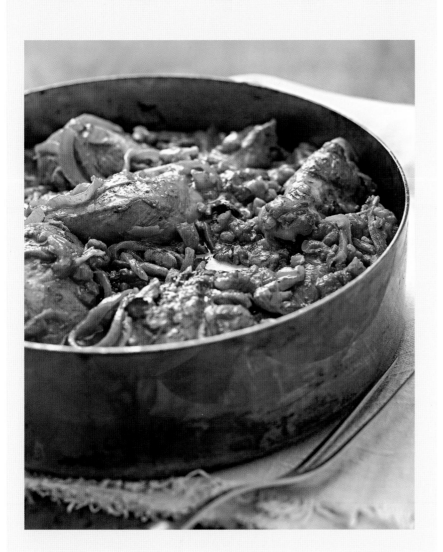

Notes from the Kitchen

- This unusual dish takes some preparation, but it is so delicious you won't mind.

- Dutch ovens are perfect for slow cooking or simmering foods. As with this recipe, adding ingredients one at a time to a Dutch oven will allow you to appreciate and enjoy the many layers of flavors.

- You can substitute 3 pounds (1¼ kg) boneless, skinless chicken breast for the whole chicken to reduce the fat content, but you may need to reduce final cooking time.

Great Herbs and Spices for Poultry

- While it's always fun to experiment with different flavors for poultry based on your own palate, here is a list of the most common, recommended seasonings to try: allspice, basil, bay leaf, bouquet garni, celery seed, chervil, chives, cilantro, ground coriander, cumin, curry powder, dill, fennel, fines herbes, ginger, green peppercorn, mace, marjoram, mustard, nutmeg, paprika, parsley, rosemary, saffron, sage, savory, tarragon, thyme, and turmeric.

Cauliflower "Cream"

A detoxifying substitute for mashed potatoes

Prep Time: 5 minutes, plus 5 to 10 minutes after cooking
Cook Time: 20 to 25 minutes

Ingredients

4 cups (940 ml) low-sodium, fat-free chicken broth (one 32-ounce or 1-L carton)

1 large head cauliflower, trimmed and cut into florets, or two 10-ounce (280-g) packages frozen cauliflower

1 clove garlic, slightly crushed

½ cup (120 ml) unflavored unsweetened almond, rice, or cow's milk (not soy milk)

2 tablespoons (28 g) butter

½ teaspoon salt

2 teaspoons (5 g) kudzu or thickener of your choice (see "Notes from the Kitchen")

2 teaspoons (5 ml) cold water

¼ teaspoon ground white pepper

¼ teaspoon onion powder

½ cup (24 g) chopped chives or finely chopped green onion (greens only, no bulb)

Few dashes hot sauce or few sprinkles paprika, optional

If using fresh cauliflower, combine the broth with enough water to fill a large pot half full and bring to a boil. Add the cauliflower and garlic and reduce the heat, simmering over medium heat until very tender, 20 to 25 minutes. If using frozen cauliflower, cook the cauliflower and garlic on the stovetop in water or broth as directed until it is very well done—fall-apart fork tender. Drain the cauliflower well, blotting with paper towels to remove any extra moisture. (This step is crucial.)

In a small saucepan, heat the milk with the butter and salt until warm (or scalded), but not boiling.

In a small bowl, mix the kudzu with the water until dissolved and add it to the heated milk mixture. Cook for about 1 minute until the mixture thickens, stirring constantly with a whisk to help prevent lumps.

In batches if necessary, put the still-warm cauliflower and garlic into blender with the warmed milk mixture. Blend until smooth. Add the pepper and onion powder and mix well. Stir in the chives or green onion and hot sauce or paprika, if using, and serve.

Yield: 6 servings

Suggested Swaps

- Simple Side: Plain Brown Rice (page 292)
- Simple Side: Spaghetti Squash (page 288)

Notes from the Kitchen

- This is a very mild dish because cauliflower can be a little bland. Punch it up with pungent flavors such as paprika, cayenne, or garlic salt to give it a little more snap.

- This dish makes a taste-comparable, low-carb, and much healthier alternative to plain mashed potatoes.

- Kudzu (kuzu) is a starchy root that is used as a thickener much like cornstarch is used for sauces, stews, and gravies. The difference is that kudzu is more nutritious and rich in protein as well as vitamins. And because of its high fiber content, kudzu also supports good digestion. Look for it in natural grocery stores or Asian markets.

Haricot Verts with Pomegranate Mint
Get your manganese here

Prep Time: 10 to 15 minutes
Cook Time: 5 minutes

Ingredients

1 pound (455 g) haricot verts, washed
  and stems removed

¾ cup (175 ml) pomegranate juice

¼ cup (60 ml) extra virgin olive oil

1 tablespoon (15 ml) lemon juice

2 tablespoons (12 g) fresh mint,
  chopped

¼ teaspoon dry mustard

Small pinch salt

1 head red leaf lettuce, washed and
  leaves separated

Extra mint leaves for garnish, optional

Suggested Swaps

- Asparagus-Endive Salad (page 206)
- Vinaigrette Salad (page 262)

Bring a large pot of salted water to a boil. Add the haricot verts, cooking until al dente, about 5 minutes.

While the beans are boiling, fill a large bowl with ice water. When the beans are cooked, pour them out into a colander, draining completely. Plunge the colander immediately into the bowl of ice water. Let the beans stand for about 5 minutes and drain again. Pat the beans dry with paper towels, transfer them to a covered dish, and refrigerate while making the dressing.

In a blender, place the pomegranate juice, oil, lemon juice, mint, mustard, and salt. Blend well until the mint is finely chopped and the dressing turns pink.

Arrange the lettuce on a large platter, placing the bottoms toward the center.

Arrange the haricot verts on top of the lettuce. Drizzle 3 to 4 tablespoons (45 to 60 ml) of the dressing over all, to taste. Store the remaining dressing in a jar with a tight-fitting lid and shake before each use. Garnish with the mint leaves, if using.

Yield: 4 to 6 servings

Notes from the Kitchen

- Haricot verts (fine green beans) are very fragile. Choose very fresh beans and cook them as soon as possible.

- If you prefer, it looks very pretty to use ½ pound (112 g) haricot verts and ½ pound (112 g) haricots blanc.

- You can substitute regular green beans for the haricot verts. However, the cook time can be longer, typically 7 to 10 minutes.

- You can freeze fresh herbs for use out of season. Rinse them, allow them to dry thoroughly, and put them between sheets of waxed paper in a resealable plastic bag or freezer storage container.

Baked Apples

An apple a day keeps heart disease away

Prep Time: 10 minutes
Cook Time: 50 minutes

Ingredients

2 tablespoons (28 g) plus 1 teaspoon
   butter, at room temperature

¾ cup (59 g) rolled oats

⅓ cup (115 g) agave nectar or ¼ cup
   (85 g) raw honey

2 tablespoons (16 g) dried sweet
   cherries or dried goji berries

¼ teaspoon salt

1 teaspoon ground cinnamon

¼ teaspoon ground nutmeg

Small pinch ground cloves

4 large firm apples, such as Pink Lady
   or Cortland

Preheat the oven to 350°F (180°C, gas mark 4).

In a small bowl, cut 2 tablespoons (28 g) of the butter into the oats, agave nectar or honey, cherries or goji berries, salt, cinnamon, nutmeg, and cloves and mix together well.

Cut one-quarter off the top of each of the apples, remove the core from the top, and chop the remainder of the tops into small pieces. Hollow cores out of the apple bottoms to form cavities in the centers, leaving the bottoms intact and discarding the cores. (A butter knife works well for this.) Mix the chopped apple pieces into the oat mixture.

Spread the remaining 1 teaspoon butter inside of the apples. Place the apples into a glass pie pan. Fill the apples with the oat mixture, pressing firmly, allowing some of the mixture to spill out over the tops. Cover the pan loosely with foil and bake for 30 to 40 minutes. Uncover and cook 10 to 15 more minutes, until the oat crumble is lightly browned and the apples are soft.

Yield: 4 to 6 servings

Suggested Swaps

• Real-Food Brownies (page 62)

• Sweet and Simple Almond Butter
  Apricot Cookies (page 168)

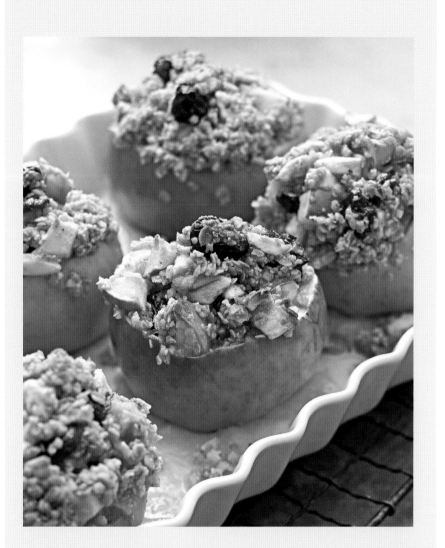

Notes from the Kitchen

- You can add ¼ cup (40 g) chopped nuts, such as almonds or walnuts, to the oat mixture.

- For a smokier, slightly bitter quality, use dried goji berries instead of the dried cherries.

- Simple baked apples actually make an excellent, sweet, high-fiber snack. Try baking them plain, cored, with no added fillers or sweeteners. Enjoy them warm or store them in the fridge for later. If you want a little more spice, try sticking 4 or 5 whole cloves into the sides while cooking. Just be sure to remove them before eating the apple!

- As a general rule of thumb, it is best to choose firm apples for baking and making pies. The best apples for baking are Rome, Jonagold, Granny Smith, Pippin, Braeburn, Northern Spy, Gravenstein, York, Cortland, Winesap, and Cameo. The worst apple for baking is the Gala. Cooking actually destroys Galas' aroma and texture!

- You can substitute Red Delicious apples for the Pink Lady or Cortland apples in the recipe. Red Delicious actually has the highest antioxidant content of all the apples, but they take longer to cook and soften than the "baking apples."

- Fall is definitely the best season for fresh apples. September through November, try to enjoy that extra freshness of apples from local apple orchards or those sold at your local farmers' markets.

Give in to a Craving? It Depends

There are two schools of thought on when you just have to have a sweet.

School number one says: Don't deny yourself. Have something good, enjoy it, and then get back on track. Try not to make it a habit.

School number two says: An alcoholic can't have a moderate amount of alcohol. Just say no. Sweets create their own cravings. It's easier to have none than to try to have a little.

I confess that I fall into both camps, though I'm more inclined to believe camp number two. That said, which school of thought is right probably depends on you. The alcoholic may not be able to have occasional alcohol, but the non-alcoholic certainly can. If you struggle with weight management issues, and you find yourself addicted to the very foods that bring you down, you're probably better off with the philosophy of school number two. Your brain doesn't process moderation. Step away from the sweets. It's easier in the long run.

But if you're okay with an occasional sweet snack or treat, and weight control isn't a big problem for you (at least not the major problem in your life), go ahead and have some sweets from time to time.

And while you're at it, consider these ideas for sweet-craving snacks that are least likely to produce out-of-control cravings of their own.

- Part-skim mozzarella stick or 1 oz cheddar with a medium apple
- Cubed Swiss cheese with berries or a small handful of dried fruit
- Apple or pear slices with nut butter
- Cottage cheese and fruit yogurt with cinnamon
- Cottage cheese with berries, apples, peaches, etc., sliced almonds, and cinnamon
- Rice, almond, soy, or low-fat cow milk and high fiber cereal or oatmeal with sliced almonds.
- Plain yogurt sweetened with agave nectar, or xylitol. Add granola, almonds, berries, peaches, dried fruit, wheat germ, ground flaxseed (like Barlean's Forti-Flax), or any high fiber cereal
- Smoothies—see chapter 14 for suggestions

Chapter 8 **Pantry List**

FOOD GROUP	FOOD
Dairy	Butter
Grains	Rolled oats
Herbs/Spices/Condiments	Black pepper Cinnamon (ground) Cloves (ground) Garlic Hot Sauce Mint (fresh) Mustard (dry) Nutmeg (ground) Onion powder Paprika Salt White pepper
Miscellaneous	Agave nectar (or raw honey) Blackstrip molasses Broth (chicken) Kudzu Olive oil (extra virgin)
Nuts/Seeds	Almond milk (or rice or cow's milk) Walnuts (or pecans)
Poultry	Chicken
Produce	Apples Cauliflower Cherries (dried sweet, or dried goji berries) Chives (or green onion) Haricot verts Lemon juice Lettuce (red leaf) Onions Pomegranate juice Tomato sauce

Clockwise from top left:
Asparagus-Endive Salad, Portobello
Buffalo Tenderloin, Silken Chocolate
Parfaits, Fragrant Chard

CHAPTER 9

Natural Protein Power

Portobello Buffalo Tenderloin

MEAL:

202 Portobello Buffalo Tenderloin

204 Fragrant Chard

206 Asparagus-Endive Salad

208 Silken Chocolate Parfaits

THIS IS A REALLY INTERESTING meal for a number of reasons. Onions and garlic, which are both members of the allium vegetable family and rich in a whole pharmacy of compounds with health benefits, have supporting roles in three of the four dishes. In addition, the meal is chock-full of spices and flavorings known for their medicinal properties, such as ginger and cinnamon.

Plus, the meal features a nice mix of protein from animal and plant sources, and last—but most definitely not least—the side dish is built around one of the most impressive vegetables on the planet (more on that in a moment).

THE ALLIUM ADVANTAGE

In Vidalia, Georgia—home of the Vidalia onion—they consume tons of onions, and the death rate from stomach cancer is 50 percent lower than in the rest of the country.

A study published in the *Journal of the National Cancer Institute* demonstrated a connection between eating onions (and other members of the allium family such as green onions, garlic, and leeks) and a significantly lower risk for prostate cancer. And onions have also been shown to have a protective effect on esophageal cancer.

Why so much cancer-fighting power? We don't know for sure, but one theory is that onions contain a compound called diallyl sulfide, which increases the body's production of an important cancer-fighting enzyme, glutathione-S-transferase.

Onions, which you'll enjoy in both the **Portobello Buffalo Tenderloin** and **Fragrant Chard**—along with garlic, which is also featured throughout this meal—contain a whole pharmacy of compounds, including sulfides, sulfoxides, thiosulfinates, and other sulfur compounds. (The sulfur is responsible for the smell.) Onions also contain powerful antioxidants and anti-inflammatories. One in particular is the superstar flavonoid called quercetin whose anti-inflammatory résumé is so strong that it can even help relieve asthma and hay fever. Quercetin also has anticancer properties of its own. And as if all that weren't enough, onions are one of a very select group of foods that—in combination—were found in one major study to reduce mortality from coronary heart disease by a very impressive 20 percent. (In case you're wondering, the others were broccoli, apples, and tea, which are all featured throughout this book.)

Here's one more wonderful thing about onions: The Environmental Working Group, a consumer protection nonprofit group, considers onions one of the twelve foods least contaminated with pesticides.

The other member of the allium family that's featured throughout this meal is garlic. You may know garlic as the favorite food of vampire fighters everywhere, which of course it is, but truth be told it's a whole lot more than its movie reputation would have you believe. Well over 1,200 pharmacological studies have been conducted on garlic, and the vast majority have indicated that this is a highly beneficial food. It's lowered serum cholesterol (and more important, it's lowered LDL—the so-called bad cholesterol) without lowering protective HDL

Save Some Green(s)

Try to use up your green veggies as quickly as possible, because their nutritional value decreases fairly rapidly over time. These veggies, like all fresh produce, will lose their valuable nutrients at a faster rate when their surrounding temperature increases. Hence, refrigerate them! Keep in mind, though, that your fridge will slow down this process, but it won't stop it.

More than half of those wonderful B vitamins and carotenoids are lost by day eight of refrigerated storage. And if you've already done some "prep work" to your greens, such as chopping or cutting, their nutrients will deteriorate even quicker.

Here's a great tip within this tip: Never store fruits that ripen alongside of your green leafies. The ripening fruit emits ethylene that will cause your greens to prematurely turn yellow and begin making those nutrients disappear. And of all the many, many types of produce, the ones that lose their nutrients the quickest are—yup, you guessed it—those green leafies!

cholesterol levels at all. It's lowered levels of triglycerides, an independent risk factor for heart disease. And it has antiplatelet activity, meaning it helps keep platelets in the blood from sticking together, helping to prevent clot formation in the blood vessels.

And there's way more to garlic than lowering cholesterol. According to Matthew Budoff, M.D., who's doing some important work in researching garlic, garlic also lowers blood pressure and helps regress plaque. Budoff explained to me in an interview that garlic also lowers homocysteine. I've written about homocysteine before, notably in *The Most Effective Natural Cures on Earth*. Homocysteine is a nasty little amino acid in the blood that, when it builds up, seriously increases your risk for three major diseases or events: stroke, cardiovascular disease, or Alzheimer's disease. We can bring homocysteine down with three simple B vitamins—folic acid, B12, and B6—but according to Budoff, garlic also helps accomplish this important task. "There's pretty consistent evidence that garlic consumption does improve your cardiovascular health," Budoff told me.

Much like with onions, compounds in garlic have demonstrated what's called chemoprotective action, meaning they're helpful weapons in the arsenal against cancer. One study demonstrated the ability of aged garlic extract to inhibit the proliferation of colorectal cancer cells. And studies show that where consumption of garlic is high, risk for stomach and colon cancer is low.

While we're on the subject of pungent spices, flavorings, and add-ons, let's not forget ginger, which is featured in the Asparagus-Endive Salad. Ginger is known in Indian medicine as the "universal remedy." It soothes an upset stomach, helps end nausea, stimulates saliva, and helps digestion. And the active ingredients in ginger—gingerols, shogaols, gingerdiones, and zingerone—are all powerful antioxidants, helping to protect cells against damage done by free radicals. At the Deepak Chopra Center, they routinely give ginger to people with cold hands and feet because of its ability to improve circulation.

AWESOME ASPARAGUS

The main ingredient in the **Asparagus-Endive Salad**—asparagus—has an interesting reputation throughout the world. In traditional Indian medicine, it's believed to help develop peace of mind, a loving nature, a good memory, and a calm spirit. The Chinese traditionalists believe it will increase feelings of compassion and love. And in the Western world, it's long been touted as an aphrodisiac. (Interestingly, asparagus is known in India by the name shatavari, which means "she who possesses 100 husbands.") Tradition and reputation aside, asparagus has a very favorable ratio of potassium to sodium. It contains folate, which is a very important B vitamin that helps prevent neural tube defects and helps reduce a harmful blood chemical called homocysteine. Asparagus is also high in vitamin K, which is essential for healthy clotting and strong bones. And a cup of asparagus also provides a decent amount of fiber (3.6 g to be exact), all for a ridiculously low number of calories—40! And speaking of fiber, one head of endive provides a whopping 16 g of the stuff, plus a surprisingly high 6 g of protein, all for a measly 87 calories. What a nutritional deal!

A WILD CHARD

Although it's a side dish, chard, which is front and center in **Fragrant Chard**, is such a spectacular vegetable that it's like the starlet that stole the movie from the above-the-title movie star. One measly cup of Swiss chard gives you almost twice as much potassium as a banana, not to mention 10,000 IU of immune-boosting vitamin A. On top of that, it offers a whopping 19,000 mcg of lutein and zeaxanthin, two members of the carotenoid family that are getting significant attention for their ability to protect the eyes and guard against vision problems such as macular degeneration. Plus you could probably feed a whole village on the stuff for fewer calories than one Big Mac. A cup of chard has … are you ready? … 35 calories. Period.

Raw Cacao versus Processed Cocoa Powder

"Chocolate is good for you!" Sounds like a line from Woody Allen's classic movie *Sleeper*, but it's actually a statement filled with truths. The catch here is that we're talking about the cacao bean, from which chocolate is made, not the processed cocoa powder found in cans.

Research shows that cacao beans contain hundreds of amazing compounds, including magnesium, iron, calcium, polyphenols (antioxidants), serotonin (an antistress neurotransmitter), and tryptophan (an amino acid that helps in the war against depression). In fact, scientists at Cornell University found that raw cacao has more antioxidants than both red wine and green tea.

Of course, this is quite different from those commercial brands of cocoa powder that we're so familiar with. You know, the cans most people reach for when baking or making hot chocolate. This stuff has reportedly been defatted, treated with alkalis, and subjected to high heat or chemicals. Yuck.

Meal Prep Tips

- The Asparagus-Endive Salad needs to chill for at least 4 hours or overnight, so make it 1 day ahead.

- Make the Silken Chocolate Parfaits first and set them aside.

- Prepare the Portobello Buffalo Tenderloin, set it to cook, and begin preparing the Fragrant Chard 20 minutes before the roast is ready to serve.

Leanest Cuts of Beef

- The leanest cuts of beef are:
  - Top round steak
  - Eye of the round
  - Top round roast
  - Sirloin steak
  - Top loin steak
  - Tenderloin steak

- Keep in mind that fat content varies with different cuts of meat and with grade. Look for USDA Choice or USDA Select grades of beef rather than USDA Prime, which usually has more fat content. Remember to trim the fat on all meats and to avoid meat that is marbled in appearance, because it has a higher fat content.

- Beyond beef, poultry is always a good option, especially white meat from the breast of chicken or turkey without the skin. Although skinless dark meat is leaner than some cuts of beef or pork, it has nearly twice the fat calories of white meat.

THE BENEFITS OF BUFFALO

As red meat goes, buffalo is a really good option. To the best of my knowledge, buffalo meat is never factory farmed. It has less fat than turkey and chicken. Buffalo spend their lives grazing on natural grasses, and it's almost a point of pride in the buffalo industry that they never use antibiotics, steroids, or growth hormones. (Of course, there might be some exception to this rule somewhere, but that has been my experience with buffalo for as long as it's been available.) Because buffalo are grass fed, buffalo meat has higher omega-3 content than ordinary supermarket ground beef, which has practically none. And the tenderloin used in this entrée is really exceptionally delicious.

WE ALL SCREAM FOR TOFU

In addition to featuring protein in its main course, this meal also features protein—tofu—in its dessert: **Silken Chocolate Parfaits**. Also known as bean curd, tofu is made by coagulating soy milk and then pressing the resulting curds, much like making cheese from milk. Tofu is usually pretty bland, but the good thing about it is that it takes on the flavor of whatever you prepare it with. It's a dietary Forrest Gump!

Another superstar ingredient in this dessert is cinnamon. This warming spice contains phytochemicals such as eugenol and geraniol, which have antimicrobial activity that can help stop the growth of bacteria and fungi. Cinnamon also contains anti-inflammatory compounds, and best of all, it can help keep blood sugar under control.

In these delicious parfaits, Jeannette has surrounded tofu with an all-star cast of mouthwatering healthy ingredients, including avocado, coconut oil, and cacao, the essence of chocolate that you read about in the introduction to this book. The result is a silken chocolate mousse that sounds almost as delicious as it tastes!

Enjoy!

Five Great Uses for Tofu

1. Use silken tofu as a high-protein "cream" base for puddings, mousses, or "cream" pies. Tofu is essentially flavorless and will take on the taste of whatever you mix it with, such as chocolate, lemon, or lime.

2. Cube very firm tofu into small chunks and add it to your vegetarian chili.

3. Drain firm tofu well (see "Notes from the Kitchen" on page 209), slice it into thin bricks, marinate it overnight in any strong meat marinade (try a teriyaki, zesty lemon, or smoky barbecue), bake it, and serve for a tasty vegetarian entrée.

4. Add silken tofu to your smoothies in place of protein powder for a thicker, creamier texture.

5. Use silken tofu as a salad dressing base in place of mayonnaise or oil for a higher-protein, lower-fat option.

Portobello Buffalo Tenderloin
An omega-3 omnibus

Prep Time: 10 minutes
Cook Time: 40 to 50 minutes

Ingredients

2 tablespoons (28 ml) butter or
    extra virgin olive oil

2 cloves garlic, minced

½ cup (50 g) green onions, roots
    removed and thinly sliced

3 portobello mushroom caps, sliced

½ cup (120 ml) red wine

1½ pounds buffalo tenderloin, trimmed
    of fat and silver skin

Garlic salt or sea salt

Ground black pepper

3 slices non-nitrate turkey bacon

Preheat the oven to 300°F (150°C, gas mark 2).

In a medium skillet over medium heat, melt the butter or heat the oil. Add the garlic and onion and sauté for 1 minute. Add the mushrooms and heat through for another 1 to 2 minutes. Add the wine and simmer until all of the liquid is dissolved.

Butterfly the tenderloin and gently stuff it with the mushroom mixture. Secure with soaked toothpicks (see "Notes from the Kitchen") and place in a roasting pan, cut side down. Sprinkle the outside with salt and pepper and wrap with the bacon. Cook for 30 to 45 minutes, or to desired degree of doneness, but don't let the internal temperature reach higher than medium (160°F [71°C]). The best practice for a slow-cooked roast is to remove it at 3° to 5° lower than your desired temperature and let it rest for 10 to 15 minutes, because it will continue to cook for a short period of time.

Yield: 6 servings

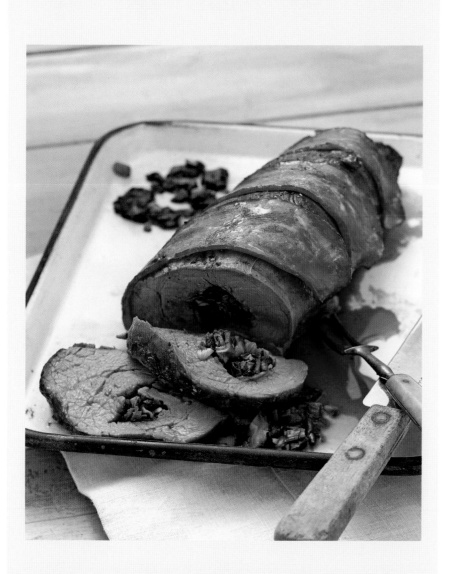

Notes from the Kitchen

• Buffalo is best cooked medium-rare to rare. The more well-done it is, the drier the meat will become. The key to roasting buffalo well is to cook it slowly, at slightly lower temperatures than beef. Because of buffalo meat's high myoglobin content, it's darker red than beef. When buffalo is cooked to medium doneness, it looks like rare beef. Use a meat thermometer to determine relative doneness because while beef and buffalo look different when cooked, their internal temperatures should be the same.

• Here's how to butterfly and stuff a tenderloin. Place the tenderloin on a piece of waxed paper (or plastic wrap). Holding a sharp chef's knife parallel to the cutting board, slice through the meat, leaving a half inch (1 cm) connected on the opposite side. Open the tenderloin like a book. For thicker cuts of meat, you can cover it with more waxed paper (or plastic wrap) and gently pound with a meat mallet or small skillet until it is about one half-inch (1 cm) thick. Spread the filler mixture in a thick ribbon down the center (the spine of the book) and roll the meat up to create a long cylinder. Secure it with toothpicks soaked in water for 10 minutes or tie it with kitchen string. Place in roasting pan, cut side down, and cook through.

Fragrant Chard

Get your potassium with Swiss chard

Prep Time: 10 minutes
Cook Time: 10 minutes

Ingredients

3 tablespoons (45 ml) roasted (or regular) almond oil

1 medium white onion, roughly diced

3 cloves garlic, crushed

1 pound (455 g) green or mixed-color chard, washed and cut into 2-inch (5-cm) pieces

¼ cup (60 ml) vegetable (or low-sodium fat-free chicken) broth

In a large sauté pan over medium-high heat, heat the oil. Add onion and sauté gently until softened but not browned, about 3 minutes. Add the garlic and mix it with the onion, cooking just enough to soften the garlic flavor, about another minute. Add the chard and turn it gently to mix it with the oil, onion, and garlic. Add the broth and cover the pan. Reduce the heat to low and simmer until the chard is al dente, for 4 to 6 minutes. Serve immediately.

Yield: 4 servings

Suggested Swaps

- Cauliflower "Cream" (page 184)
- Roasted Rutabaga Chips (page 128)

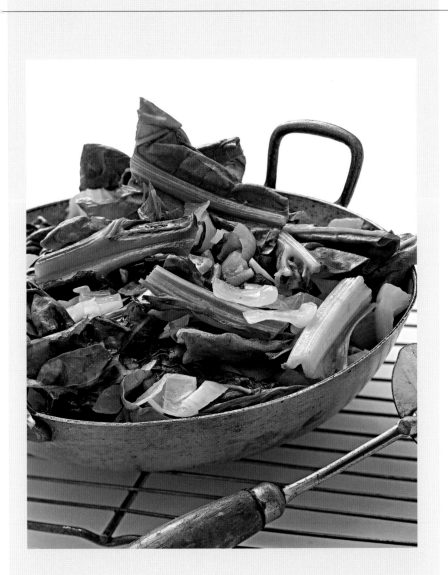

Notes from the Kitchen

- Swiss chard—like spinach, beets, and rhubarb—contains compounds called oxalates, which may be a problem for people who have a certain type of kidney stone called calcium oxalate stones, which are formed from a combination of calcium and oxalate. This is not a problem for most people, however.

- Roasted almond oil, which is available at gourmet markets, has a slightly nuttier flavor than raw almond oil, but the effect is subtle so they can easily be exchanged.

- Instead of vegetable broth, you could use the liquid from a jar of roasted red peppers.

- Chard is done when the bitter taste is gone but it is not yet soggy.

- This side dish also works cold as a salad. Try it with a garnish of sliced peaches or tomatoes. Or serve it as a main dish with beans. Try it with Peruano beans (a sweet, creamy, pale yellow bean) for something a little different.

Asparagus-Endive Salad

Low-cal freshness from the garden

Prep Time: 5 to 10 minutes
Cook Time: 10 minutes, plus 4 hours or overnight chill time

Ingredients

1½ pounds (680 g) thin asparagus

1 8-ounce (225-g) can sliced water
  chestnuts, drained

¼ cup (60 ml) almond oil

½ cup (120 ml) white wine vinegar

½ cup (120 ml) water

¼ cup (85 g) blackstrap molasses

1 teaspoon ground ginger or
  ginger juice

1 teaspoon finely grated onion

½ teaspoon salt

½ teaspoon lemon zest

1 large head endive

Cherry tomatoes, halved, optional

Watercress or parsley, optional

Trim and rinse the asparagus.

In a large pot fitted with a steamer basket, steam the asparagus until tender-crisp and bright green, for 3 to 8 minutes, depending on the freshness and thickness of the stalks.

Transfer the asparagus to a colander and pour cold water over it for a minute or so. Drain well and pat dry. Transfer the asparagus to a large bowl and let it cool for a few minutes. Toss the cooled asparagus with the water chestnuts and oil and set aside.

In a small saucepan, combine the vinegar, water, molasses, ginger or ginger juice, onion, and salt. Heat to boiling and remove from the burner. Cool it for 10 to 15 minutes, then pour it over the asparagus mixture. Sprinkle with the lemon zest and cover. Refrigerate for at least 4 hours or overnight. Drain.

Separate the endive leaves and arrange them on a platter. Place 2 or 3 asparagus spears onto each endive leaf. Garnish with the cherry tomatoes and watercress or parsley, if desired.

Yield: 6 servings

Suggested Swaps

- Haricot Verts with Pomegranate Mint (page 186)

- Caesar Salad (page 294)

Notes from the Kitchen

- Asparagus is a versatile vegetable. While its true growing season is spring, you can find it in most grocery stores year-round. It can be served hot, cold, or at room temperature.

- Fresh, tasty asparagus is bright green with firm stalks and compact tips. Thinner stalks are generally more tender than the thicker ones. The freshest asparagus has firm, straight stalks and closed, compact tips.

- To trim asparagus, bend it gently. If it's fresh, it should naturally break off at the point where the woody portion meets the more tender stalk. For very thick stalks, you may need to peel the tougher outer skins off with a vegetable peeler. Thicker stalks require more cooking time.

- To make ginger juice, peel and grate fresh ginger, then squeeze the juice out of the gratings. You'll need about 2 tablespoons (16 g) of gratings to get 1 tablespoon (15 ml) of juice.

Silken Chocolate Parfaits

A sweet indulgence that won't raise your blood sugar

Prep Time: 15 minutes plus 20 minutes to drain the tofu (optional) and soak the dates
Cook Time: None, but with optional overnight refrigeration

Ingredients

⅓ cup (25 g) pitted dates

1 pound (455 g) firm silken tofu

4 tablespoons (32 g) raw cacao or high quality cocoa powder

3 tablespoons (60 g) agave nectar

2 teaspoons (10 ml) coconut oil, warmed to liquid

¼ teaspoon cinnamon

1 teaspoon vanilla extract

1 small, very ripe soft avocado

5 cups (550 g) fresh berries such as raspberries or 6 cups (1020 g) strawberries, rinsed and dried, and sliced if using strawberries

2 small ripe bananas, peeled and thinly sliced

Mint leaves, optional

Crushed roasted nuts, such as toasted almonds, cashews, or chestnuts, optional

Measure the dates into a glass measuring cup and cover with warm water to 2 inches (5 cm) over the tops. Mix the dates around with the water so they are all are in contact with the water. Let the dates sit for 20 minutes (or up to an hour) and drain off the soaking water.

Pour off the water from the tofu.

In a food processor, puree the tofu, dates, cacao, agave, coconut oil, cinnamon, and vanilla, scraping down the sides of the bowl frequently, for 2 to 4 minutes, or until smooth.

Cut the avocado in half, remove the pit and peel, cut away any knots, and add half of it to the food processor. Store the other half with the pit for another use later. (The pit helps slow the browning process.) Blend together all of the above ingredients well, scraping down the sides of the bowl several times, until the mix is silky smooth with no lumps.

Cover the bottoms of 6 glasses with a layer of the berries. Cover the berries with a thin single layer of the banana. Spoon ⅙ cup (38 g) of pudding over the banana. Repeat the layers and top with the last few remaining berries. Serve at once with the mint or nuts, if using, or chill overnight.

Yield: 6 servings

Suggested Swaps

- Real-Food Brownies (page 62)
- Sweet Potato Pie with Almond-Oat Crust (page 236)

Notes from the Kitchen

- This dish is beautiful in parfait glasses. But if you don't have them, use 6 short glasses that hold about 1 cup of liquid.

- You will need approximately ¾ cup (95 g) of berries, ⅓ of a banana, and ⅓ cup (77 g) of pudding for each parfait.

- If you wish, you can omit the bananas. Their main purpose in this recipe is visual aesthetics: to keep the parfait layers separate. But of course they add lots of nutrition as well.

- If you simply pour the liquid off the tofu, as described in the recipe, you will get a softer, more liquid pudding. For a stiffer, drier consistency, drain the tofu instead. To drain silken tofu, make a hammock out of cheesecloth, bundle the tofu inside, and tie it to the faucet of your sink for 20 minutes. All of the excess water will drain away. If you have no cheesecloth, you can also use the weight method, although it works better with nonsilken varieties: Drain the standing water from the tofu and pool the tofu on a plate. Cover the tofu with a second flat plate and carefully place 2 cans of soup or beans on the upper plate. Allow the tofu to drain in the sink for 20 minutes. Tip off the excess water, and the tofu is ready.

- You can use very ripe avocados for this recipe, but keep them warm when ripening: Cold makes them blacken and turn stringy. (See "Citrus Avocado Salad with Nut Oil" on page 38 for more on using avocados.)

- You can experiment with other extracts, such as orange, hazelnut, or even coconut.

Energy, Protein, and Health Bars—What's the Real Deal?

Once upon a time there were PowerBars. You had to try ten stores to find one that carried them, and they came in one flavor. They were advertised as being for athletes and had a vaguely healthy reputation.

Not any more. PowerBars, along with about twenty-five (when I last counted) competitors, now have their own section in virtually every grocery store and even in the same gas station and convenience stores, which used to feature only Slurpees, candy bars, and chips. Known variously as energy bars, nutrition bars, or protein bars, they're part of a category called meal replacements that's one of the hottest areas in the food industry.

But are these things any good? Depends. Good meal replacement bars seem to fall into two overall classes—the boutique ones made from nothing but real foods, such as fruit and nuts, and the more manufactured, mass market bars that contain protein (whey or soy) and other ingredients. The ones that are made from real foods (like LaraBars, for example) have lots of nutrition, but are also very high in natural sugars, which can be a problem for many people. They also tend to be low in protein.

In an ideal world, you'll want to see ingredients that are real, like almond butter, nuts, or fruit, i.e., ingredients that you actually recognize. Though some bars meet that criteria, even a cursory reading of labels shows that many bars don't come close. If it's full of ingredients you can't recognize or pronounce, don't eat it. And if it contains any trans fats or high fructose corn syrup, don't even consider it!

So what's the take-away message? The nutritional content of bars varies widely and what suits one person just fine might not be the best choice for another. Athletes on the go can easily do with higher carbohydrate bars, but their needs are going to be different from the average sedentary office worker who just wants a healthy afternoon snack.

Bottom line: look for commercial bars that have higher fiber, lower sugar, no trans fats, and some protein. Read the label and don't be fooled by the name or packaging.

Chapter 9 **Pantry List**

FOOD GROUP	FOOD
Dairy	Butter (or extra virgin olive oil)
Herbs/Spices/ Condiments	Black pepper (ground) Cinnamon (ground) Garlic Garlic salt (or sea salt) Ginger (ground or juice) Lemon zest Mint leaves Salt Vanilla extract Watercress (or parsley) White wine vinegar
Meat	Buffalo tenderloin
Miscellaneous	Agave nectar Blackstrap molasses Broth (chicken or vegetable) Cacao or cocoa powder Coconut oil Red wine Silken tofu Water chestnuts
Nuts/Seeds	Almonds (or cashews or chestnuts) Almond oil
Poultry	Turkey bacon
Produce	Asparagus Avocado Banana Chard (green or mixed colors) Cherry tomatoes Dates (pitted) Endive Onions (green and white) Portobello mushroom caps Raspberries (or strawberries)

Clockwise from top left:
Holiday Waldorf Salad; Citrus-Stuffed Herbed Turkey; Sweet Potato Pie with Almond-Oat Crust; Roasted Brussels Sprouts, Asparagus, and Broccoli with Toasted Hazelnuts; Cranberry-Orange Relish

Healthiest Holiday Meal

Citrus-Stuffed Herbed Turkey

MEAL:

224 Citrus-Stuffed
Herbed Turkey

230 Roasted Brussels
Sprouts, Asparagus,
and Broccoli with
Toasted Hazelnuts

232 Holiday Waldorf Salad

234 Cranberry-Orange
Relish

237 Sweet Potato Pie with
Almond-Oat Crust

WHEN I was the iVillage.com weight loss coach, each holiday season I received hundreds of questions on my message board about holiday eating. How to do it. How not to do it. Specifically, how to avoid the five to ten pounds that thousands of people gain between late autumn and early January and that few ever take off again. Is there a secret?

Well, no. Except to maybe try not to put the weight on in the first place.

Holiday time is a wonderful time of celebration, reunion, family, and—hopefully—gratitude. And unfortunately, overeating. It's kind of built in to the season. But there are a lot of really smart things you can do to minimize the damage, both to your health and to your waistline. First and foremost: Eat meals like this holiday feast Jeannette put together, which provides an amazing cornucopia of nutrients and—for a holiday feast—an amazingly low amount of sugar. As for the rest of the things you can do, I've put together some of my favorite tips for holiday eating.

Meanwhile, let's get to the food!

JUSTIFICATION TO EAT DESSERT FIRST

I can't help myself; I have to start with the dessert.

If you're going to eat dessert—and who isn't around holiday season?—this is the way to go. You'll love the **Sweet Potato Pie with Almond-Oat Crust**. Sweet potatoes are delicious in a variety of settings (including, by the way, as snacks, cold, right out of the fridge), and they are by far the most nutritious of all potatoes. Most orange foods contain a lot of either vitamin A or members of the carotenoid family or—as in the case of sweet potatoes—both. In this case, one medium potato has more than 21,000 IU of immune-supporting vitamin A and a nice hefty dose—more than 13,000 mcg—of beta-carotene. Plus there's almost 4 g of fiber per potato, and more potassium than a banana. Not bad for the basis of a dessert!

To make the pie filling, you add to the sweet potatoes a couple of eggs, which are long one of my most favorite perfect foods for their combination of protein, good fat, eye-supporting carotenoids, and brain-supporting choline. Though Jeannette mentions one of the nonhydrogenated margarines as a possible shortening, I have no problem with butter, but I recommend you get it from organic or grass-fed sources, in which case butter can be a really fine food. (It made the cut in my book *The 150 Healthiest Foods on Earth*!)

The pie filling is naturally sweetened by a combination of orange juice and agave nectar. Agave nectar, which is also called agave syrup, is similar to honey but thinner, so it flows more easily. (There's a dark kind and a light kind; the dark is less filtered, so a little richer in nutrients.)

The agave plant contains plant chemicals such as saponins and inulin. Saponins are natural detergents that are found in a lot of desert plants and may have some health benefits in humans. They bind to cholesterol and may help lower it. Other even more important benefits of saponins are being explored in research. In one Canadian study, saponins had an inhibitory effect on the growth of human carcinoma (cancer) cells in a test tube. And inulin is a type of fiber that actually serves as a probiotic, meaning it is food for the good bacteria in your gut.

Don't misunderstand. You're not going to get a ton of health benefits by using a little agave syrup as a sweetener, even though the actual agave plant does contain these beneficial compounds. And the syrup is hardly calorie-free. But the point is that as baking sweeteners go, this one has a pretty darn good pedigree, and it beats the heck out of the usual granulated sugar that's used in recipes like this one.

Meal Prep Tips

- Holiday prep can be crazy-making. To enjoy your holiday meal, plan with some care.

- Make the Sweet Potato Pie with Almond-Oat Crust one day ahead or first thing the morning of your meal.

- Make the Cranberry-Orange Relish the morning of your meal.

- Begin the Citrus-Stuffed Herbed Turkey prep five to six hours before you want to be sitting down to eat.

- Prepare the Roasted Brussels Sprouts, Asparagus, and Broccoli with Toasted Hazelnuts one hour before the end of the turkey cook time and slip them into the oven when you remove the turkey to rest.

- Make the Waldorf Salad right after the veggies go in to roast.

Urban Legend: The Turkey Made Me Sleepy

Many people believe that the reason they get so sleepy after a big holiday meal containing turkey is that turkey contains tryptophan, which is an amino acid that the body uses to make serotonin, a brain chemical involved in promoting feelings of calm and relaxation.

It's true that tryptophan does make you sleepy. In fact, it was at one time very popular as a sleeping aid. And it's also true that turkey does contain tryptophan. But it's a pretty small amount; no more than many other protein sources. Besides, for tryptophan to have that kind of an effect you'd have to take it alone on an empty stomach. And you'd have to take a lot more than is found in turkey.

So it's an urban legend that the tryptophan in turkey makes you sleepy. What really makes you sleepy is overeating. Tons of calories, many of them from sugar, drive blood sugar up and then way back down again, making you feel like a zombie. Blood is diverted from the extremities (and the brain) to the digestive system to handle the load. No wonder you doze.

Falling asleep before the dishes get washed has absolutely nothing to do with tryptophan. Sorry. And by the way, how many beers did you have with that meal again?

There was some discussion among "Team Jonny" about the use of flour in this recipe (and some others), so here's the deal: We decided that the amount used here is not going to kill you. All the other ingredients are terrific—we're talking, after all, about making a pie, and there's just not much you can do without at least a small amount of the stuff. Do I love the idea of flour in general? Of course not. But let's get real. We're making a holiday meal and it includes pie. All things considered, this is a great recipe, and while it might not be perfect, I think the amount of flour we needed to include to make it come out right is ultimately a pretty minor problem as far as your overall health goes. And guess what? You can avoid the whole issue by making it crustless; it tastes absolutely great that way! (See "Notes from the Kitchen" on page 237.)

THE NEW WALDORF SALAD

The Waldorf Salad was created by Oscar Tschirky, the maitre d'hotel (not the chef) at the famed Waldorf Astoria hotel in New York, in 1896. It was an instant hit back then, and this version—**Holiday Waldorf Salad**—will be an instant hit in your kitchen more than a century later.

If you're new to the Waldorf Salad, you'll be certain to remember this one. The classic Waldorf had apples, celery, raisins, walnuts, and mayo as key ingredients; later versions added all kinds of spices, yogurt, orange juice, grapes, pears, dates, and even Cajun seasoning. Jeannette's version is classic, simple, delicious, and healthy. Based around apples and celery, it substitutes yogurt for the mayo, sweetens with a little honey and orange, and spices up with ginger, walnuts, cranberries, and grapes. You also have the option of adding cherries, figs, or dates. It's loaded with phytochemicals from the fruit, plus fiber from the apples, and—if you use the walnuts—some omega-3 fats. And … it's beyond delicious.

What traditional holiday meal is complete without cranberry sauce, here jazzed up in **Cranberry-Orange Relish**? The little berries possess anticancer properties, inhibit the growth of common pathogens and microbes, and are well known for having antibacterial properties that aid in the prevention of urinary tract infections.

Because of their high vitamin C content, cranberries have one of the most potent antioxidant résumés of any fruit, and they can act as a great preventive against atherosclerosis. They are best known for their usefulness in treating urinary tract infections because the acidity of cranberry makes the urine more acidic and kills the infection. Another way they work is by inhibiting the adhesion of bacteria to the mucosal wall of the gastrointestinal tract, thereby preventing the bacteria like *H. pylori* and *E. coli* from "sticking," growing, and proliferating.

Cranberries even have bioactive compounds that have been found to be toxic to a variety of cancer tumor cells. It's actually a shame that we don't eat them on a regular basis and save them only for special holiday meals, when a lot of the stuff we normally eat is half cranberry, half sugar. But not the special Cranberry-Orange Relish featured in this meal. You'll get all the health benefits of real cranberries, sweetened only with a little honey or agave nectar and flavored with orange. What could be better?

BROCCOLI AND BRUSSELS SPROUTS: VEGETABLE ROYALTY

Before getting to the main course (did you notice we're kind of working backward here?), let's talk for a minute about the vegetable side dish, **Roasted Brussels Sprouts, Asparagus, and Broccoli with Toasted Hazelnuts.** Earlier (see page 155), I talked about what I call the royal family of vegetables, the Brassica family. The head of this family (no pun intended) is cabbage, but every member of this family contains cancer-fighting indoles as well as other phytochemicals that are a boon to your health. And two of the stars of this royal vegetable dynasty are found in this wonderful side dish: broccoli and Brussels sprouts.

Broccoli and Brussels sprouts both contain a family of anticancer phytochemicals called isothiocyanates, which fight cancer by basically neutralizing carcinogens (cancer-promoting chemicals). Isothiocyanates have been shown to inhibit tumors and also to help prevent lung and esophageal cancer. Broccoli in particular contains a potent isothiocyanate that acts as an inhibitor of mammary tumors.

Broccoli also contains a compound called indole-3-carbinol, which is a strong antioxidant and stimulator of detoxifying enzymes that also acts as a traffic cop for estrogen, moving it along down the paths where it is least likely to be carcinogenic.

Choosing a Turkey

I've written elsewhere in this book (see page 179) and extensively in *The 150 Healthiest Foods on Earth* about why I believe organic, free-range meat is the best kind to buy, and all of that applies to turkey as well. You're less likely to get a dose of antibiotics, steroids, and hormones with your meat when you buy birds that have been raised humanely and allowed to eat their natural diet. It's that simple. If you're going to eat meat, which is an individual choice, I hope you'll buy the best you can possibly afford. The difference is worth it.

Brussels sprouts contain a chemical called sinigrin that suppresses the development of precancerous cells. When sinigrin breaks down, it creates a chemical called allyl isothiocyanate, which is the compound responsible for the characteristic smell of Brussels sprouts. But allyl isothiocyanate also persuades precancerous cells to commit suicide—a process called apoptosis.

And both Brussels sprouts and broccoli are high in a special superstar plant chemical called sulforaphane that helps increase the production of enzymes that "disarm" damaging free radicals and help fight carcinogens.

To this dynamic duo, Jeannette has thrown in some asparagus, which is a nice little low-calorie, high-potassium vegetable that is also is high in vitamin K, a lesser-known vitamin that's essential for strong bones and healthy clotting. Add some heart-healthy olive oil, some immune system –strengthening garlic, and hazelnuts—which bring fiber, minerals, and healthy monounsaturated fat to the party—and you've got an absolutely smashing side dish that will make you feel virtuous just for looking at it, let alone eating it!

TERRIFIC TURKEY

Then there's the main course--What else? Turkey, delicious in the **Citrus-Stuffed Herbed Turkey**. Turkey is a good source of protein, has some nice minerals such as potassium, and is fairly low in calories. Turkey is also low in fat, and most of the fat it does have is either monounsaturated or polyunsaturated. Even the dark meat has only a couple of grams of saturated fat per serving, which is nothing to worry about.

When you surround that succulent turkey with the outstanding Roasted Brussels Sprouts, Asparagus, and Broccoli with Toasted Hazelnuts, toss in the scrumptious Holiday Waldorf Salad, and garnish with the antioxidant-rich Cranberry-Orange Relish, you've truly got a holiday feast. And you get to top the whole thing off with one of the best desserts on the planet—Sweet Potato Pie with Almond-Oat Crust.

Enjoy!

Ten Tips for Cooking Healthy over the Holidays

Here are some of our best suggestions for making holiday food even healthier!

1. Replace some butter with some olive oil, for a better balance of healthy fats. Try a 50/50 mix.

2. Replace heavy carbs such as potatoes and stuffing with herbs that can flavor up a turkey or vegetables.

3. Go organic to avoid hormones, pesticides, and antibiotic residues in meat or produce.

4. Replace mayonnaise with low-fat yogurt for tasty dressings without the extra fat and artificial stuff. (Note: There's nothing wrong with mayonnaise, especially homemade from real eggs, but you'll save some calories this way.)

5. Trim all visible fat from meats. Stick with lean cuts and white meat.

6. Consider more nutrient-dense foods for desserts such as sweet potatoes, pecans, and pumpkin. You'll feel better about doing a little overindulging if the choices are healthier.

7. Check ingredients on any cans that you use. High-fructose corn syrup can reside in any package or can, and it is certain to be in canned cranberries. Avoid the bad sugars and look for fresher ingredients.

8. When choosing honey, try to find raw, unfiltered, cold-pressed organic honey. (See "Notes from the Kitchen" on page 233.)

9. Don't overdo the number of courses. Stick with a few basics for a satisfying meal that doesn't overstuff your guests.

10. Consider serving a salad as the last course (or dessert).

Seven Tips for Holiday Eating

Wonderful as holidays may be for everything else, they can be downright deadly for sticking to a weight loss plan.

Because holiday eating can mean so many things—family stuff, office parties, special desserts, and the inevitable boxes of cookies at the water cooler—it's hard to come up with one surefire strategy that will work for everyone in all situations. One strategy, however, will invariably make a difference no matter what the particulars of the situation: rehearsal.

Most of us know what we're going up against. For some it's the sight of the holiday table and relatives you haven't seen all year. For others, it's virtually everyone in the office bringing in their aunt's special Christmas cookies. For still others it's the stress eating associated with the mixed emotions of family reunions and juggling even more commitments than the usual overload. Even vacations can be stressful, and if they happen to involve airports at holiday time it's a no-contest. Add it up and you've got a potential disaster. In fact, forget the "potential" part. You're looking at emotional and physical overload, and what that means for your waistline (let alone your sense of well-being) is not good.

Rehearsing a problem situation in your mind before it happens helps you to arm yourself with strategies, visualize yourself doing them, and experience the positive results. That way you're not caught unprepared, and you can actually practice reacting to a variety of dangerous situations.

That's what coaches do with their athletes; it's what boxing trainers do with their fighters. "When he throws that left hook, you step in under and throw a right to the body." Studies have shown improvement in sports performance just through visualization exercises, in which, for example, basketball players mentally "practice" shooting baskets under various conditions. You can do the same thing with the holidays.

Of course, to do this effectively, you have to be clear on what you want to happen. That's why I like using a tool I call the "proactive food journal." Here's how to do it: Pick a day, visualize what it's going to be like, where you're going to be, and with whom. Think about what food is likely to be available, when you're likely to be hungry, and what the circumstances are going to be. (Is your Aunt Tina going to be there insisting you try her special key lime pie? Are you going to be in a restaurant known for its crème brûlée and homemade breads? Are you going to be in a fast-food restaurant taking care of six kids? Is the sister whom you hate going to be there silently judging everything you eat?

Now write down what you're going to eat. Decide in advance, early in the day or even the night before. Visualize the situation. If there's temptation or anxiety, close your eyes and picture it. Hear in your mind's ear what people will say. See yourself responding in a way that would make you proud of yourself. That might be allowing yourself one or two bites of something "off your diet," or it might mean being spartan. The point here is not what you choose, but that *you* choose it.

And that you then stick to it. As Sondheim wrote, "The choice may have been mistaken. The choosing was not." The point here is to put *you* in charge of what happens, not the circumstances.

If you can accomplish that, you have begun a journey that will help you manage your weight, and one that will empower you in all areas of your life.

Here are seven tips on how to use visualization to help you with holiday eating.

1. Close your eyes and really picture the situation clearly.
2. Ask yourself whether what's being offered is going to be something that supports you in what you're doing or takes you off course.
3. Decide what you wish to allow yourself to indulge in—if anything—and when you decide to do it, indulge in it with gusto.
4. Make the choice and take the action.
5. Don't arrive hungry. A cup of soup or vegetable juice before arriving at a big event will help keep you in charge of your own actions.
6. Remember that stress leads to stress eating. Stress management is a critical part of managing weight gain during the holiday season.
7. If you do indulge, for goodness' sake enjoy it!

Safety First

The Food Safety and Inspection Service recently changed the recommendations for how high a temperature cooked poultry should be cooked to. Previously, experts recommended cooking whole turkeys to 180°F (82°C) and turkey breasts to 170°F (77°C). The new cooking recommendation is 165°F (74°C) for both. Check the internal temperature in the innermost part of the thigh and wing and the thickest part of the breast with a meat thermometer.

Citrus-Stuffed Herbed Turkey

A bounty of protein and potassium

Prep Time: Overnight to brine, overnight again for optional drying, and 30 minutes to prepare for cooking.
Cook Time: 3 hours and 45 minutes to 4 hours and 15 minutes, plus 20 minutes to rest before carving

Ingredients

Brining Solution

You will need 2 to 3 gallons (8 to 12 L) of brining solution for an 18- to 20-pound (8- to 9-kg) turkey.

Per gallon (4 L) of water:

1 cup (300 g) sea salt or kosher (not table salt)

½ cup (170 g) raw honey

2 teaspoons (4 g) finely grated lemon peel, optional

2 teaspoons (4 g) orange peel, optional

½ tablespoon cardamom pods, optional

1 teaspoon dried thyme, optional

Turkey

1 18- to 20-pound (8- to 9-kg) free-range, not self-basting, turkey

8 sprigs each of fresh rosemary (young and tender, not woody), sage, and thyme (or other herbs of your choice), rinsed and lightly dried (should total 1¼ to 1½ cups or 55 to 90 g when coarsely chopped)

2 shallots, peeled and halved

1 whole head garlic, peeled and crushed

1 lemon

1 orange

4 tablespoons (½ stick, or 55 g) butter, softened

2 tablespoons (28 ml) extra virgin olive oil

Salt

Ground black pepper

½ cup (120 ml) sherry

Starting with 2 gallons (8 L) of water, mix the brining solution in your roasting pan by combining all ingredients in correct proportions and stirring until the salt and honey are dissolved.

Rinse the turkey in plain water and pat it dry. Place the turkey in a lobster pot or large stockpot. (You can also use a plastic bucket if you line it with 2 or 3 clean garbage bags.) Pour in the brining solution to cover the turkey. If you need more brine to completely immerse the turkey, mix up another gallon. Place the turkey in the refrigerator for 12 to 24 hours. Remove the turkey from the brine, rinse very well under running water to remove all the brine, and dry thoroughly, including the cavity. (See "Notes from the Kitchen" on page 228.)

Preheat the oven to 400°F (200°C, gas mark 6).

Stem and coarsely chop the herbs, setting aside about three-quarters of them (⅔ to 1 cup or 40 to 60 g of herbs). Mince the remaining one-quarter (about ½ cup or 30 g) and put into a medium bowl. Add the shallots and garlic.

Quarter but do not peel the lemon and orange and squeeze them gently to make a little juice, tossing the fruit and juice together with the herb mixture.

In a small bowl, using your hands, mix the butter with the oil until creamy. Moving carefully so as not to puncture the skin, work your hand between the turkey skin and the breast as far as you can go to create a pocket over both breasts. Smear half of the butter-oil mixture over the breasts, covering as much meat as you can reach. Place half of the reserved, coarsely chopped herbs (or whole sprigs, see "Notes From the Kitchen" on page 228) in each pocket (on top of each breast). Do this carefully and when complete, gently reshape (from the outside) the herb "pouches" above each breast to look rounded and smooth. Salt and pepper the inside of both cavities and stuff them with the fruit and herb mixture. Tuck the wings behind the back, tuck the skin folds over the cavities to close, and truss the legs. Smear the entire bird with the remaining butter-olive oil mixture and sprinkle with salt and pepper. Slowly pour the sherry inside of the breast pockets, working it around to the leg joints.

Place a V rack inside of a roasting pan and cover it with foil. Poke about 15 holes into the foil. Place the turkey on the V rack, breast side down. Bake for 45 minutes, then reduce the oven temperature to 325°F (170°C, gas mark 3). Turn the turkey bird breast side up, baste (you can supplement the juices with a few tablespoons of sherry if you wish), cover with foil, and continue to cook for 2½ to 3 hours more, depending on the size of the turkey.

Remove the foil to brown the breast and continue to cook for another 30 to 40 minutes, or until the thickest part of the breast and innermost parts of thighs and wings register 165°F (74°C) on a meat thermometer. (When the turkey is done, the legs should roll loosely on the joint, and the leg juices should run clear.)

Let the turkey rest on a cutting board for about 20 minutes before carving.

Yield: For turkeys weighing more than 12 pounds, allow ½ to ¾ pound (225 to 340 g) per person, so an 18-pound (8-kg) turkey can serve between 24 to 36 people (photo page 226)

Notes from the Kitchen

- People tend to go overboard with amounts and number of dishes in a holiday meal. There's really no need for this. Try serving just the four basic courses in this simple, elegant, and nutritious meal. No one will complain.

- Finding a free-range turkey for Thanksgiving may not be as easy as you might think. "Free-range" simply means that the birds have access to the outside, but many don't make it out to graze and roam because of the crowded conditions and other inhumane practices used to guarantee quick-growing, profitable turkeys in time for the holidays. So it's worth the effort to shop around. We recommend two websites for more information: www.localharvest.org and www.slowfoodusa.org. Both can point you in the direction of local farmers who live by a philosophy of clean, delicious organic turkeys that are raised in humane conditions.

- Brining, a very simple process, improves the quality of the cooked turkey. The combination of the salt and sugar helps the cells of the meat to both open and retain moisture, creating a juicier end product. You can experiment with adding different herbs and spices to the mixture, such as cinnamon sticks, whole peppercorns, or try a fresh bunch of thyme instead of the dried. Also, some people like to use apple cider in place of half of the water.

- If you brine the turkey right before cooking, the skin will not become as crisp because it will "steam" during cook time. If you want a crisper skin, brine the day before, rinse the turkey as directed, and place it uncovered, breast side up, in the basting pan overnight in the refrigerator. This allows the excess moisture to evaporate, and you will get a crispier skin when it's cooked.

- Most fresh organic turkeys do not come self-basted. If you manage to find one, it's probably brined in table salt, complete with iodine load, which is not great for the meat, and white sugar. This is not terrible, it's just much poorer quality.

- If you are working with a large bird (that will take a longer cooking time) or desire a milder herb flavoring, use the whole sprigs (without chopping) under the skin. Just remove the large pieces when the cooking is complete and use them as a garnish.

- If you don't own a V rack, try using 2 miniature loaf pans (4 or 5 inch × 3 inch, 10 or 13 × 8 cm) face down and set on either side of your roasting pan (in the middle, lengthwise). If using the loaf pans, no need for tinfoil over the "rack."

- This type of whole-bird preparation typically calls for a stick or more of butter. Consider using half butter and half extra virgin olive oil, as we have done here, which introduces some mono-unsaturated fat.

- Here's how to carve a turkey:

1. Place the turkey on a cutting board with a trough to catch the juices. Cut through the crispy skin that connects the leg and the breast and slice down, pulling the thigh away from the bird. Continue until you reach the joint and cut through it to separate the leg.

2. Carve off the breast meat in one piece: Slide the knife along one side of the breastbone, as close to the bone as possible. Cut the breast off the carcass.

3. Place the breast meat on the cutting board and thinly slice. Transfer the meat to a platter.

4. Place the leg on the board and cut through the joint between the thigh and drumstick. Transfer to the platter. Detach the wing where it connects to the bird. Transfer it to the platter, then repeat.

- By avoiding the typical stuffing, mashed potatoes, and gravy fillers in this healthier turkey dinner, you are eliminating a significant portion of the fat, not to mention reducing the number of calories from simple carbohydrates that often load up holiday meals. The herbed meat of this turkey is so flavorful that you won't miss a thing!

- Don't throw the turkey carcass away! Once you've eaten most of the meat, save the skeleton and remaining meat bits to make a turkey broth for fabulous soup. If you've had it with turkey for the moment, freeze it for a couple of weeks and make turkey soup as a warming winter treat.

Roasted Brussels Sprouts, Asparagus, and Broccoli with Toasted Hazelnuts
A healthy harvest of cancer prevention

Ingredients

1 pound (455 g) Brussels sprouts

1 or 2 whole peeled cloves garlic, halved if they are large

2 teaspoons (10 ml) plus 1 tablespoon (15 ml) extra virgin olive oil

Salt

Ground black pepper

1 pound (455 g) thin asparagus spears

2 to 3 large crowns broccoli

¼ cup (60 ml) Minus 8 (or balsamic) vinegar

¼ cup (35 g) hazelnuts, lightly roasted and coarsely chopped

Suggested Swaps

- Wild Rice and Green Beans with Shiitake Sauté (page 82)
- Fragrant Chard (page 204)

Prep Time: 20 minutes
Cook Time: About 25 minutes

Preheat the oven to 375°F (190°C, gas mark 5).

Stem the Brussels sprouts and cut them in half, quartering any large ones. Place them into a medium bowl. Add the garlic and 2 teaspoons (10 ml) of the oil and season lightly with the salt and pepper.

Spread the Brussels sprouts in a single layer in a small baking span and roast for 10 minutes.

Meanwhile, trim the asparagus. Remove the tough lower stems from the broccoli, peel off the tougher stem skin with a paring knife, and slice the stalks lengthwise into long strips from stem through florets. Toss the asparagus and broccoli gently in a bowl with the remaining 1 tablespoon (15 ml) of the oil and light salt and pepper until coated.

Spread the asparagus and broccoli on a second baking sheet, sized to fit in the oven with the first.

After the Brussels sprouts have roasted 10 minutes, add the broccoli-asparagus pan to the oven, and continue to roast for about 15 minutes longer until all vegetables have softened, turned bright green, and lightly browned.

Meanwhile, warm the vinegar in a small saucepan and simmer lightly until it begins to reduce and thicken slightly.

When vegetables are complete, remove the garlic and blend it with the warm vinegar in a blender.

Arrange the vegetables on 2 serving platters, with the broccoli framing the plate of Brussels sprouts and plate of asparagus. Spoon the vinegar evenly over the vegetables, sprinkle with the nuts, and serve at once.

Yield: 6 to 8 servings

Notes from the Kitchen

- Always roast or toast nuts and seeds at relatively low temperatures because their oils are delicate. On the stovetop: Dry-sauté nuts in a pan on medium-low. In the oven: Spread a single layer of nuts on a baking sheet and roast in a warm oven (350°F, 180°C, gas mark 4) for just a few minutes for seeds and 7 to 12 minutes for nuts. Only heat seeds until they release their oil; you can smell the change. Seeds are the most delicate; don't let them actually brown or they will turn slightly bitter. Nuts can turn a warm golden brown, but they scorch easily, so watch them closely toward the end of the cook time. Look closely at your nuts and seeds. Can you see a faint sheen developing and smell their rich aroma? Then they are almost done!

- To get the right consistency of the hazelnuts in this recipe, pound them in a paper bag with a meat mallet on your cutting board.

Holiday Waldorf Salad

A healthy, fiber-filled version of this classic dish

Prep Time: 5 to 10 minutes
Cook Time: None

Ingredients

¼ cup (60 g) plain low-fat or full-fat yogurt

1 teaspoon raw honey

3 tablespoons (45 ml) freshly squeezed orange juice

¼ teaspoon powdered ginger

2 small crisp red apples (such as Macoun or Pink Lady), cored and chopped into small pieces (about 2 cups or 300 g)

4 celery stalks, thinly sliced

½ cup (75 g) purple seedless grapes, halved, optional

¼ cup (37 g) dried cranberries or cherries or chopped figs or dates

½ cup (75 g) lightly toasted walnuts, coarsely chopped

8 cups (160 g) hearts of romaine, chopped into bite-size pieces

In a small bowl, whisk together the yogurt, honey, orange juice, and ginger.

In a salad bowl, combine the apples, celery, grapes (if using), cranberries or cherries, walnuts, and romaine.

Pour the yogurt dressing over the salad and toss all together to combine well.

Yield: 8 servings

Suggested Swaps

- Citrus Avocado Salad with Nut Oil (page 38)

- Caesar Salad (page 294)

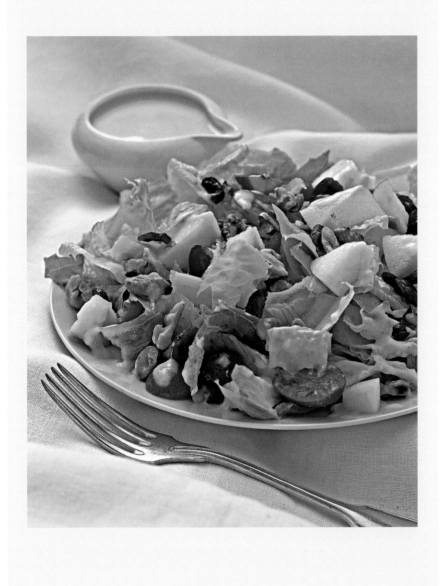

Notes from the Kitchen

- The Waldorf Salad makes a terrific dessert. Or by adding some chicken, you can make it into a main dish. It's especially great for summer lunches, and it travels pretty well in an airtight container.

- Replacing the mayonnaise with low-fat yogurt transforms this timeless dish into a healthy classic.

- Using yogurt instead of oil as a base allows you to create a myriad of tasty low-fat dressing options. Try a savory dressing with fresh minced garlic, chopped chives, lemon, and pepper.

- When choosing honey, try to find raw, unfiltered, cold-pressed organic honey. It's a whole different food from the stuff in the squeezy bear. Since the honey hasn't been processed at high heat, it still contains live enzymes. It also contains plant polyphenols that are known for their antioxidant activity and are important for human health. P.S.: Raw unfiltered honey tastes better, and it's just as sweet as the commercial stuff. Neither raw nor commercial honey spoils.

Cranberry-Orange Relish
Autumnal antioxidants

Prep Time: Less than 5 minutes
Cook Time: None, but the flavors will develop if left to sit for a couple of hours before serving

In a blender or food processor, blend together the cranberries, oranges, and agave or honey until a juicy relish is formed.

Yield: 12 to 14 servings

Ingredients

4 cups (440 g) fresh cranberries, or two 8-ounce (225-g) bags frozen unsweetened, thawed and rinsed

2 oranges, peeled and halved

⅔ cup (230 g) agave nectar or honey, or more or less to taste

Notes from the Kitchen

- Put this relish in heavy rotation on your menu of choices for meals throughout the year, not just at holiday season. Feel free to halve the recipe if you need less at one time. The relish goes well with a surprisingly wide variety of dishes, and cranberries are really, really good for you!

- If you can't find fresh cranberries, you can substitute 4 cups (440 g) dried whole cranberries, but use 4 small oranges and omit the agave/honey. Dried cranberries are almost always heavily sweetened, so this version doesn't have the crisp tartness of the fresh, but it is still better for you than the stuff in a can! Look for juice-sweetened dried cranberries only, not the sugar-sweetened varieties.

- Cranberries are delicious and nutritious, and they're also beautiful. If you wish to serve a canapé or cheese platter during a holiday gathering, fill your serving platter with a bag of fresh cranberries and place the food items on the top—lovely!

Suggested Swaps

- Raw Chocolate Fondue (page 108)
- Silken Chocolate Parfaits (page 208)

Sweet Potato Pie with Almond-Oat Crust

Rich in vitamin A and beta-carotene

Prep Time: 20 to 25 minutes
Cook Time: About 50 minutes

Ingredients

Pie Filling

3 pounds (1¼ kg) sweet potatoes (5 or 6 medium), peeled and cut into 1½-inch (4-cm) pieces

2 eggs

¼ cup (85 g) agave nectar

¼ cup (60 ml) almond milk

¼ cup (55 g) melted Natucol or Earth Balance (nonhydrogenated vegetable spread) or butter

3 tablespoons (45 ml) freshly squeezed orange juice (from about ½ orange)

1 teaspoon vanilla extract or ½ teaspoon vanilla extract and ½ teaspoon orange extract

1 teaspoon ground cinnamon

½ teaspoon ground nutmeg

¼ teaspoon ground cloves

Pie Crust

⅔ cup (54 g) whole oats, ground into flour in food processor

⅔ cup (100 g) almonds, ground into fine meal in food processor

⅔ cup (74 g) whole wheat pastry flour

¼ cup (60 ml) almond oil or grapeseed oil

¼ cup (85 g) agave nectar

¼ cup (60 ml) water

Pie Topping

1 cup (100 g) raw pecan halves or toasted sliced almonds

2 tablespoons (40 g) brown rice syrup

1 tablespoon (20 g) agave nectar

(see recipe directions on page 238)

Notes From the Kitchen

- This dish works perfectly well crustless. To avoid flour entirely or speed up the preparation time, omit the crust and bake the sweet potato filling in an 8-inch (20-cm) square glass baking dish and serve it "naked."

- Having your heavier starchy vegetables for dessert is both filling after lighter holiday fare and significantly higher in nutrients than typical fruit pies, with less than a third of the fat.

- You can replace the cinnamon, nutmeg, and cloves with 2 teaspoons of pumpkin pie spice.

(continued from page 236)

To make the pie filling: Preheat the oven to 350°F (180°C, gas mark 4).

Place the sweet potatoes in a large pot of boiling water and boil until very soft, for 10 to 12 minutes.

Meanwhile, place the eggs in a mixer and beat well.

When the potatoes are soft, drain them well and add them to the mixing bowl.

Add the agave nectar, almond milk, spread or butter, orange juice, extract(s), cinnamon, nutmeg, and cloves and mix until light and fluffy with no lumps.

To make the pie crust: Place the oats, almonds, and flour in a large mixing bowl and mix to combine.

In a small bowl, whisk together the oil, ¼ cup (85 g) agave, and water. Pour them into the oat mixture. Mix until well combined. (The batter will be sticky.)

Oil a 10-inch (25-cm) deep-dish pie plate and spread the crust mixture evenly onto plate with oiled fingers.

To make the pie topping: Place the pecans in a single layer on a baking sheet and place nuts and pie crust into preheated oven. Bake for 5 minutes and start checking the pecans, being careful not to scorch them. Remove after 5 to 8 minutes, or when lightly toasted. Remove the crust after 10 minutes.

In a small bowl, combine the brown rice syrup and 1 tablespoon (20 g) agave nectar and add the hot pecans, tossing to thoroughly coat.

Spoon the potato mixture gently into the crust and arrange the nuts on top of the filling. Bake for 30 to 35 minutes, or until the crust is lightly brown at the edges. Cool the pie for at least 20 minutes before serving.

Yield: 8 servings

Food for Thought

Fifty percent of all charitable giving is done during the holidays at the end of the year. It's a great time to remember how fortunate we are and to reach out to those who are less so. For those so inclined, here are a few ways you can make a difference this holiday season (or any other time).

Consider setting up a giving tree in your place of business. You simply contact local social service organizations, tell them you'd like to set up a giving tree, and expect them to interview kids to find out what they would most like to receive this season. Buy a live or artificial tree and place it in a well-trafficked area. Collect cards or "ornaments" that the agency will prepare containing a child's name, age and gift request, and hang those on the tree (for example: Kim, age 6, Barbie doll). Suggest that donors find a wish they'd like to make come true, purchase the gift requested, wrap it, and put it under the tree. (Make sure the request card is attached so the right gift goes to the right child.) Then just arrange for the agency to deliver the gifts to the kids, and know that you've made some less fortunate kids very, very happy.

Other charities to consider: Toys for Tots (www.toysfortots.org), Make-A-Wish Foundation (www.worldwish.org), and one of my personal favorites, Mercy Corps (www.mercycorps.org).

Local charities deliver holiday dinners to needy people in almost every city. (The New York City Rescue Mission in New York City is one, but you can easily find its counterpart in the city or country in which you live.)

What's most important is not who you give to, but that you do it.

Savory Snacks—The Satisfying and Portable Polymeal

Oftentimes you aren't in the mood for something sweet, but you're hungry and you need a pick-me-up between meals. This is the perfect time for a savory snack.

Savory snacks (and mini-meals) provide another golden opportunity to add a variety of different nutrients to your daily diet. Didn't load up on the vegetables at lunch? Now's your chance—grab a handful of rainbow-colored crudités and some zippy lemon hummus for dipping.

Or perhaps you had a light veggie-based lunch like a big spring salad, but you didn't have enough protein with it and an hour later you're hungry again: Pull out a tuna pack and enjoy it straight with a squeeze of lemon or a tablespoon of fruit-sweetened cranberry sauce (Knudsen makes one).

Nuts are a key part of the polymeal formula but they don't go easily into every meal menu. Snack time provides the perfect chance to grab a small handful. They are so rich in fiber and great fats (even a little protein) that they make an ideal stand-alone savory snack. Jeannette carries raw almonds with her everywhere she goes—they fit right into her purse!

Try these other savory snack ideas:

- Veggie sticks paired with any protein
- A part-skim mozzarella stick with carrots or celery
- Baby carrots poked into green or black olives
- Rice cakes with hummus or nut butter
- Whole wheat or rice pretzels or crackers with any nut or protein spread, meat, fish, or cheese
- Smoked fish with horseradish on whole wheat or rice crackers
- Cottage cheese with tomatoes or peppers and sea salt/pepper
- No-sugar bean dip or refried beans with baked tortilla chips or raw veggie sticks
- Salsa and avocado with baked corn chips
- Babaghanoush with veggie sticks
- Shrimp with low-sugar cocktail sauce
- Boiled egg alone or with veggies
- Non-nitrate cold cut roll-ups around veggie sticks

Chapter 10 **Pantry List**

FOOD GROUP	FOOD
Dairy	Butter, Eggs, Plain yougurt
Grains	Flour (whole wheat pastry), Whole oats
Herbs/Spices/ Condiments	Black pepper (ground), Cinnamon (ground), Cloves (ground), Garlic, Ginger (powdered), Nutmeg (ground), Rosemary (fresh), Sage (fresh), Sea salt (or kosher), Thyme (dried and fresh), Vanilla extract (or orange extract)
Miscellaneous	Agave nectar (or honey), Brown rice syrup, Minus 8 vinegar (or balsamic), Natucol (or Earth Balance or butter), Olive oil, Raw honey, Sherry
Nuts/Seeds	Almonds, Almond milk, Almond oil (or grapeseed oil), Hazelnuts, Pecans (or almonds), Walnuts
Poultry	Turkey
Produce	Apples (Macoun or Pink Lady), Asparagus, Broccoli, Brussels sprouts, Celery, Cranberries (fresh), Cranberries (dried, or cherries, figs or dates), Grapes (purple seedless), Lemon, Lettuce (Romaine hearts), Oranges, Orange juice, Shallots, Sweet potatoes

2 | One-Pot Polymeals
with Simple Sides

Clockwise from top left:
Venison Stew; Lamb Chops and
Sauerkraut; Simple Side: Vinaigrette
Salad; Simple Side: Steamed Green
Veggies and Nuts; Red Beans, Brown
Rice, and Lean Beef

CHAPTER 11

Meat One-Pots

MEALS:

256 Lamb Chops and Sauerkraut

258 Simple Side: Steamed Green Veggies and Nuts

260 Venison Stew

262 Simple Side: Vinaigrette Salad

264 Red Beans, Brown Rice, and Lean Beef

EACH OF the three delightful meals in this chapter is hearty, satisfying, and complete—minus, of course, the dessert! (But feel free to add a few squares of dark chocolate and a glass of red wine to make the evening complete.) The main one-pot meal is protein-based and relatively easy to prepare, and will feed a family nicely. Though this is the one-pot chapter devoted to meat-based dishes, you can prepare the third meal—red beans and rice—as a meatless dish. Simply leave out the beef or turkey. It still tastes great.

PROTEIN-PACKED LAMB

The first meal, **Lamb Chops and Sauerkraut**, features a meat we haven't talked about so far. Lamb is a staple in countries throughout the world, especially in the Middle East and the Mediterranean. It's also common in New Zealand and Australia. Technically the term "lamb" is reserved for the meat of a domestic sheep a year old or younger. (Older sheep are called either hogget or mutton.)

I've talked elsewhere in this book (see page 49) and also in *The 150 Healthiest Foods on Earth* about the benefits of grass-fed meat. In a perfect world, you wouldn't eat any other kind. (I know this isn't a perfect world, and if you need to eat "regular" meat, so be it, but I feel strongly about the quality of the meat we eat when we do eat meat and want to let you know why.) Point is, it's kind of moot when it comes to lamb, because lamb by definition is young (sometimes as young as one month), and it is almost always raised on pasture. And it's just not popular enough here in the United States for the big agribusinesses to have bothered to figure out a way to "factory farm" lamb. Hence it's a meat that—as far as I know—is usually free from steroids, hormones, and extra antibiotics.

Like beef, lamb is a great source of protein; one 4-ounce (115-g) loin chop has 27 g. Also like beef, only about half the fat is saturated; the other half is monounsaturated, the same kind that's in olive oil. One loin lamb chop also has about a third of the Daily Value for B12, about 40 percent of the daily value for niacin, and just under 25 percent of the Daily Value for zinc. You can get the chops in either loin or rib. The rib is a little higher in calories and fat and a little lower in protein.

AMAZING APPLES

One of my favorite superfoods in the Lamb Chops and Sauerkraut is apples. I've raved about apples earlier in this book (and, of course, in *The 150 Healthiest Foods on Earth*), but just to recap, they're loaded with an important member of the flavonoid family called quercetin, which is known for its anticancer activity as well as for being a powerful anti-inflammatory. One medium apple also has 3 g of fiber, much of it from pectin, which has been shown to lower both cholesterol and glucose (sugar) levels in humans. In a recent (August 2007) study at the University of Georgia, prostate cancer cells exposed to pectin under laboratory conditions were reduced in number by up to 40 percent. And the apples in this dish are cooked; interestingly, University of Georgia research found that the anticancer properties of pectin increased significantly when it was heated. Remember to buy organic apples, because apples are at the top of the list for heavy pesticides.

FERMENTED FOODS

Another great food in this meal is sauerkraut. It's superb, especially when it's prepared the traditional way. Why? Because it pairs cabbage—one of the healthiest foods on Earth—with one of the most healthy forms of processing on the planet: fermentation. The result is a superfood that's absolutely loaded with healthy bacteria called *lactobacillus*, which improve digestion, immune function, and the absorption and assimilation of nutrients.

I'm a huge fan of naturally fermented foods. Fermentation is an ancient technique of preparation and preservation in which food is naturally "processed" by microorganisms such as bacteria that break down the carbohydrates and protein in the food. Unfortunately, commercial food processors have tried to standardize the fermentation techniques, and many modern mass-produced foods (such as canned olives and pickles) are not actually fermented. They're just treated with chemicals, packed in salt, and canned. That's not what you want. Only authentic fermentation gives you the amazing health benefits of the live cultures such as *lactobacillus*, which offer wonderful benefits to the immune system and to digestion. These live cultures also help control inflammation, which is a central feature of so many degenerative diseases, including heart disease. And active cultures can actually suppress *H. pylori*, which is the type of bacteria responsible for most cases of ulcers.

Besides having the advantages of containing live cultures, sauerkraut also brings to the table all the wonderful nutritional and health benefits found in the original food used to make it—cabbage. I've written elsewhere (see page 155) about the amazing benefits of cabbage (and its relatives in the Brassica family), but just to remind you, cabbage is high in a group of plant compounds called indoles that have demonstrated anticancer activity. Cabbage plus fermentation equals a health bonanza.

Another supporting player in this one-pot cast of characters is leeks, which add a delicious flavor to the mix and also contain a whole pharmacy of compounds with health benefits, including thiosulfinates, sulfides, sulfoxides, and other sulfur compounds. The active substances in leeks, including allyl sulfides, help provide protection against cancers by blocking the action of hormones or chemical pathways within the body that promote cancer. Regular consumption of allium vegetables—the family to which leeks belong—is associated with a reduced risk of both colon and prostate cancers.

VENISON: NO NEED TO HUNT FOR ITS MINERALS

Okay, I feel exactly the same way you do. Tell me "venison," and I think "Bambi."

I remember many conversations about venison back during the twelve years I was the iVillage.com weight loss coach. Whenever anyone would mention eating venison, I'd cringe, until one of my valued and respected message board moderators finally did the cyber equivalent of "pulling me aside" and explained that she—and many people across the country—hunt and eat deer for food, not for sport. She explained that where she came from, people relied on deer to provide meat throughout the winter, freezing the steaks, and living on them for months. Her attitude toward these gorgeous animals was similar to that of the Native Americans. She respected and appreciated the animals that gave their lives so that she and her family could eat. She too loved Bambi, but deer was an important part of her diet.

I admit it, I'm still a bleeding-heart liberal, but I've come to appreciate what an amazingly healthy and nutritious meat venison is. It's even

Great Herbs and Spices for Red Meat

Beef: Bay leaf, bouquet garni, caraway seeds, chives, cinnamon, coriander (ground), cumin, fennel, green peppercorn, horseradish, mace, marjoram, mustard, oregano, paprika, savory, and thyme

Lamb: Allspice, basil, coriander (ground), fines herbes, marjoram, mint, mustard, oregano, parsley, rosemary, sage, savory, and tarragon

Venison: Bay leaf, caraway seeds, fines herbes, ginger, green peppercorn, horseradish, juniper berries, mace, marjoram, mustard, sage, and savory

Braising and Healthy Cooking

Braising is a cooking method usually used for tougher cuts of meat, such as pot roasts, rumps, shanks, and ribs, and sometimes for vegetables. The food cooks in liquid, similar to stewing, which results in very tender meat. For best results, make sure that each piece of meat, or vegetables that you are braising, is similar in size. Most braised dishes take from 45 minutes (for smaller cuts of meat and poultry) to 6 hours (for really tough shanks and ribs). Here's how to do it.

1. Heat a little oil in a heavy frying pan.

2. Season the meat or vegetables with salt and pepper, or with whatever seasonings you will be using.

3. When the pan and oil are hot, add the meat or vegetables and sauté them at medium-high—hot enough to brown the meat but not hot enough to destroy the essential fatty acids in the oil. This will add color and flavor.

4. Once browned, add enough liquid to the pan to come about halfway up the sides of the meat or vegetables. Liquid used for braising is usually water, stock, wine, or a combination.

delicious in recipes like this **Venison Stew**. Venison is packed with protein, vitamins, and minerals, such as phosphorus, potassium, zinc, and iron. And if it's caught in the wild, venison is free of antibiotics and synthetic hormones.

Venison also has less fat and calories than beef. According to Charles J. Alsheimer in the September 2000 issue of *Deer & Deer Hunting*, deer accumulate most of their fat around their organs and in single layers, typically atop muscle and underneath the hide. These fat layers can be easily removed during the butchering process. Whitetails also have less fat in their muscle tissues because they are constantly exercising. Indeed, all cuts of deer meat are extremely low in fat.

My friend Regina Wilshire, N.D., who contributed this recipe and many ideas for this book, is responsible for the suggestion that we use a couple of tablespoons of flour in this venison recipe. Here's why: The flour acts to protect the meat from forming nasty compounds appropriately nicknamed AGES, which stands for advanced glycation end-products. AGES result from protein being browned or caramelized when it comes into contact with high-sugar or carbohydrate foods. (Nutritionist Heather MacLean Walters, Ph.D., wrote an entire book on the health dangers of AGES, interestingly called *The Body Browning Effect*.) So that's why the flour is there. Thanks, Regina.

PRODUCE POWER

If you're familiar with my previous writing or with my philosophy about food and health at all, you probably know I'm no fan of potatoes. So no one was more surprised than I was when I recently read that Agricultural Research Service plant geneticist Roy Navarre, Ph.D., and his colleagues at Washington State University and Oregon State University identified sixty different kinds of phytochemicals and vitamins in the skins and flesh of 100 wild and commercially grown potatoes. According to Navarre, the number of phenols, which are plant chemicals with health benefits, found in red and Norkotah potatoes rivals that of broccoli, Brussels sprouts, and spinach. I'll be honest: I'm not completely convinced—yet. But at least I don't feel so bad about including potatoes in the Venison Stew one-pot meal. Besides, I never said they didn't taste great.

Also featured in the stew's cast of ingredients are our old healthy staples onions and garlic, which are both members of the allicin family, and both foods that have consistently been associated with reduced rates of cancer and heart disease. Add in the mushrooms and spices and you're good to go. According to Wilshire, calorie for calorie crimini mushrooms are superdense with nutrients, providing selenium, riboflavin, copper, niacin, pantothenic acid, phosphorus, and zinc. They're ridiculously low in calories, so by definition they can't provide a lot of all those nutrients, but the calories they do contain are far from empty!

BEANS AND RICE: PERFECTLY COMPLETE

Our third one-pot meal can be a chameleon. You can make **Red Beans, Brown Rice, and Lean Beef** with beef, turkey, or no meat at all. Like the old commercials for breath mints ("two, two, two mints in one!"), it's a double bargain: a protein-packed vegetarian meal or a traditional meat-based dish. Either way it's hearty, satisfying, and nutritious.

Like all beans, red beans are fiber heavyweights. High-fiber diets are associated with lower risk for a host of diseases, including heart disease and diabetes. As I've said many times before, Americans just don't get enough of this important dietary necessity. All the major health organizations recommend between 25 and 38 g of fiber a day. Our Paleolithic ancestors got at least 50 g a day, but today the average American gets about 8. Not good. Just recently, researchers from the University of Massachusetts Medical School found that people eating a high-fiber diet were 63 percent less likely to have elevated levels of C-reactive protein, a measure of inflammation that can be an independent predictor of both diabetes and heart disease. Beans are a superb way to get fiber in your diet, and this one-pot dish is a great way to eat beans!

5. Lower the heat and let the recipe simmer slowly or place the whole pan (ovenproof, of course) in the oven and bake it. Do not allow the liquid to evaporate.

6. If you want to use the braising liquid as a sauce, leave the pan uncovered so moisture can evaporate, thus concentrating the flavors. If you wish, add other ingredients to flavor the liquid along the way, such as vegetables or herbs and spices. Also, only do this with cuts that take less than 90 minutes or so to cook. Otherwise, just cover the pan.

7. When you're braising, make sure the liquid level doesn't get too low, or you'll be baking and not braising. On the other hand, make sure the liquid level doesn't get too high. If the liquid covers the meat and vegetables entirely, you'll be stewing and not braising. Either way, the results will be totally different.

For years we've heard about the "complete" protein formed by rice and beans. Here's the story: Protein is actually made up of molecules called amino acids, of which there are about twenty that are used by the cells to assemble proteins in the body (like muscles, bones, neurotransmitters, and hormones). These amino acids are conventionally divided into two groups: essential and nonessential. The terminology is misleading because all amino acids are essential and important. Many of them can be made in the body from other molecules, and they're called nonessential. Those that can't be made in the body from other molecules are called essential, meaning it's essential that we get them from the diet.

When nutritionists talk about a "complete" protein, they mean a protein that provides all of the essential amino acids. Most vegetable sources don't, though there are exceptions, such as spirulina and quinoa. But by eating a variety of vegetable sources, you can get all the essential amino acids. Rice and beans is the most typical example of a combination that provides a "complete" protein from plant sources.

Nutritionists have debated for decades about how to rate different kinds of protein for quality. Many believe that only animal foods provide the highest-quality protein, and there's some data to back that theory up. However, other compelling data shows that you can get all your amino acids from vegetable sources. You can avoid the whole debate by using both! This dish is equally tasty with some beef or turkey, but if you prefer, you'll get a fine amount of protein with just the rice and beans. Your choice.

Most people believe that white rice is the least "good" of the rices, being a basically nutritionally empty food with little fiber or nutrients. But unfortunately the differences between the rices are not as great as we'd like to think. All the rices are pretty high on the glycemic rating, meaning they raise blood sugar fairly quickly (not a good thing). But when you mix rice with beans, vegetables, and the optional meat, the glycemic impact of the meal is substantially blunted, and the impact on your blood sugar much more moderate. Neither brown nor white rice is a vitamin heavyweight. Where brown rice edges out white is for fiber. Brown rice has 3.5 g of fiber per cup, as opposed to a measly 1 g for white rice. Many Eastern cultures highly value rice as a gentle and natural detoxifier. It is very easy to digest, especially if well chewed, and when eaten in small amounts over time is said to calm and soothe the digestive system.

Our old friends onion and garlic add cancer-fighting plant compounds, and the olive oil provides heart-healthy monounsaturated fat. Tomatoes, especially when cooked, provide lycopene, which is an important antioxidant and member of the carotenoid family. The red bell pepper is rich in vitamins C, A, and K and the mineral potassium, as well as a super member of the carotenoid family—beta-cryptoxanthin—which may lower the risk of developing lung cancer. And the hot pepper is also rich in nutrients, plus it contains an active ingredient called capsaicin that enhances circulation and may also help aid digestion. And capsaicin depletes something called substance P, a chemical that transmits pain messages to the brain.

Even the oregano used for seasoning in this dish is a health food! According to some research, it has forty-two times more antioxidant activity than apples, thirty times more than potatoes, twelve times more than oranges, and four times more than blueberries. Plus the essential oil of oregano contains two compounds—thymol and carvacrol—that have antifungal, antibacterial, and antiparasitic properties, and one compound—rosmarinic acid—that has antimutagenic and anticarcinogenic properties. It's no wonder Cass Ingram, D.O., called his book about oregano *The Cure Is in the Cupboard!*

To each of the one-pot meals, don't forget to add the greens, and have a square of dark chocolate on me!

Enjoy!

The Best Way to Cook Game Meat

Whether you are cooking venison, buffalo, or some other type of exotic game meat, keep in mind that the meat will naturally be leaner—and therefore tougher—than farm-raised fatty cows and chickens, so cooking temperatures and seasonings will vary. Venison, buffalo, and elk have the consistency of beef but a lot less fat and therefore must be cooked medium to medium-rare.

Here's how.

First, trim off as much fat as you can, because fat is one of the factors that gives game meat that "gamey" taste. For cooking quickly, sear the meat on both sides at a high heat (just enough to brown the sides). Next "lard it" by placing bacon over the top of it, which will keep the juices in, then cover it and place it in the oven. (If the taste of bacon seems too strong, other options for larding are butter and olive oil, which will also seal in juices.) Cook the meat until the internal temperature reaches about 135°F (57°C). Anything higher than that will dry out the meat and turn it to leather.

If you are slow-cooking the game, season it first with whatever you'd like, but leave out the salt, because that will dry out the meat. Lard it again with a few strips of bacon and place it in the oven at about 225°F (107°C). Let the meat cook for 8 to 16 hours. This process will produce a very tender piece of game meat.

Lamb Chops and Sauerkraut

Powerful protein and a cancer-fighting sidekick

Prep Time: 15 minutes
Cook Time: 4 hours (on high); 6-7 hours (on low)

Ingredients

6 to 8 small loin or rib lamb chops,
  ½ inch (1 cm) thick

1 teaspoon almond oil

2 medium leeks

3 cups (675 g) sauerkraut, drained

¾ cup (175 ml) low-sodium
  fat-free chicken broth

⅛ teaspoon garlic powder

1½ teaspoons caraway seed

½ teaspoon thyme

½ teaspoon salt

¼ teaspoon ground black pepper

2 apples, cored and sliced

Trim all of the visible fat off of the edges of the lamb.

In a skillet, heat the oil over medium-high heat. Carefully pour or wipe excess oil from the pan. Briefly sear each side of the lamb and set aside.

Cut most of the tough greens off the tops and about ½ inch (1 cm) of the bulb off the bottoms of the leeks. Slice the leeks lengthwise down the middles and cut them into 1-inch (3-cm) sections. Immerse the leeks in a sink of water and separate them to clean thoroughly. Drain the leeks and place them in a slow cooker, covering the bottom.

In a small bowl, whisk together the sauerkraut, broth, garlic powder, caraway seed, thyme, salt, and pepper. Pour half of the mixture over the leeks. Place the lamb on top and pour the remaining half of the mixture over the lamb. Top with the apple.

Cover the slow cooker and cook on low for 6 to 7 hours or on high for 4 hours.

Yield: 4 servings

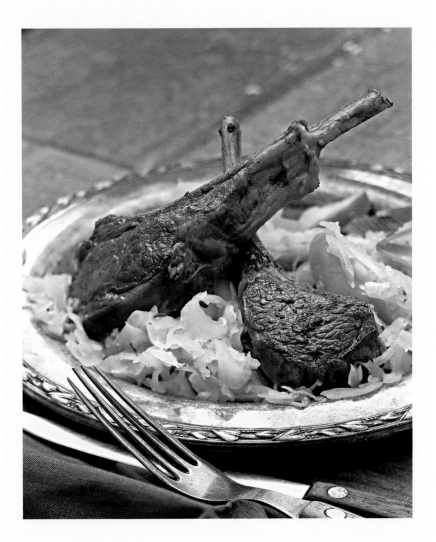

Notes from the Kitchen

- In the past, you could only buy fresh lamb during the spring or summer; hence the term "spring lamb." But because lamb is now available year round, the term "spring lamb" doesn't mean much anymore.

- Lamb is very perishable. Honor the "use-by" date, keep it in the original packaging until you use it to minimize exposure to air, and keep it cold or frozen.

- Brown the lamb chops first on the stovetop to give them a nice seared surface, because that won't happen in a slow cooker. It's not quite as important for skinned poultry, but it really helps the flavor of red meat cuts.

- If you freeze lamb, make sure to wrap it tightly. With proper freezing, it should keep for at least a few months.

- Loin lamb chops are less fatty than rib chops. Two chops generally yield about 4 ounces (115 g) of lean meat. Lamb has less marbling than other red meats, so if you trim the visible fat on the outside of the chops, you'll remove most of it from the cut.

Steamed Green Veggies and Nuts

A frenzy of folate and good fat

Prep Time: 5 to 10 minutes
Cook Time: 3 to 10 minutes

Ingredients

4 cups (280 g) asparagus, young green beans, or broccoli florets, washed and trimmed

¼ cup (30 g) dry-roasted nuts, chopped, such as almonds, walnuts, or pecans

Fit a large pot with a steamer basket, pour water into the pot to just under the basket line (so it doesn't come in direct contact with the veggies), and bring the water to a boil. Add the vegetables and steam until bright green and tender-crisp, for 3 to 10 minutes. Sprinkle the nuts over top and serve.

Yield: 4 servings

Notes from the Kitchen

• Steaming plain green vegetables is a wonderful, simple way to prepare them. The light cooking brings their color up and makes them easier to digest. To steam green vegetables, place a steamer basket in a large saucepan with water to just under the basket line (so it doesn't come into direct contact with the veggies). Bring the water to a boil and place the washed, trimmed vegetables in the basket. To retain more nutrients, cook them for the shortest amount of time. Broccoli can be ready in about 3 minutes, thin asparagus in about 6 minutes, and very fresh green beans in about 7 to 10 minutes. In general, the older or thicker a vegetable is, the longer it will need to steam properly.

Ingredients

3 pounds (¼ kg) venison, cut into
   1½- to 2-inch (4- to 5-cm) chunks

2 tablespoons (15 g) whole wheat flour

1 teaspoon salt, plus more or less to
   taste, divided

1 teaspoon ground black pepper, plus
   more or less to taste, divided

5 tablespoons (70 g) butter, divided

1 teaspoon dried thyme

2 tablespoons (28 ml) extra virgin
   olive oil

2 onions, finely chopped

2 large cloves garlic, minced

½ cup (120 ml) dry white wine

1½ cups (355 ml) low-sodium
   beef broth

⅓ cup (80 ml) Worcestershire sauce

1 tablespoon (5 g) lemon zest

1 bay leaf

1 cup (180 g) tomatoes, seeded, peeled,
   and coarsely chopped

1 cup (130 g) baby carrots

1 pound (455 g) small red baby
   potatoes, halved

1 pound (455 g) fresh whole crimini
   mushrooms

¾ cup (33 g) frozen green beans or
   baby peas, thawed

2 tablespoons (8 g) fresh parsley,
   chopped

Venison Stew
Lean protein and nutrients galore

Prep Time: 20 minutes
Cook Time: 1 hour 30 minutes

Preheat the oven to 500°F (250°C, gas mark 10).

Pat the venison dry with paper towels.

Place the flour, salt, and pepper to taste in a resealable plastic bag. Place the venison in the bag and toss to coat with the flour.

In a heavy cast-iron skillet, heat 3 tablespoons (45 g) of the butter until bubbling, then add the venison 6 or 7 chunks at a time. Brown the venison carefully on all sides, then transfer it to a 4- to 5-quart (4- to 5-L) Dutch oven. When all of the venison is browned, discard the browned butter, wipe the skillet, and set it aside.

Toss the thyme with the venison. Place the Dutch oven, uncovered, in the oven and cook the venison, turning once after 5 minutes, for about 10 minutes, or until the meat is slightly crusted. Remove from the oven and reduce the oven heat to 325°F (170°C, gas mark 3).

In a skillet, heat the oil over low heat. Add the onions and cook for 5 minutes. Add the garlic and cook for about 5 minutes more, or until the onions have softened and browned a bit. Increase the heat to high. Add the wine and broth and bring to a boil. Boil for 3 minutes, then pour into the Dutch oven over the venison. Add the Worcestershire sauce, lemon zest, bay leaf, 1 teaspoon salt, and 1 teaspoon pepper and toss together.

Add the tomatoes, carrots, and potatoes and toss together. Cover the Dutch oven and bake on the middle shelf of the oven for 1 hour, or until the venison is fork-tender.

While the stew is cooking, melt the remaining 2 tablespoons (28 g) butter. Add the mushrooms and toss them in the butter, turning them frequently with a spoon until tender, about 10 minutes.

(continued on page 261)

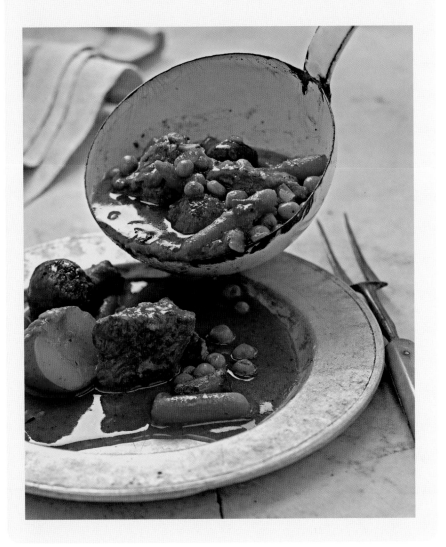

Notes from the Kitchen

- This Venison Stew takes some time and attention, but the layered cooking techniques and richness of the resulting flavors nicely mellow any gaminess of the venison.

- As an alternate to the red potatoes, try using 1½ cups (350 g) butternut squash cut into 1½-inch (4-cm) cubes, roughly the size of the potatoes.

- If you aren't in a hurry, another way to efficiently defat a stew sauce like this one is to put the separated sauce and stew into the refrigerator overnight. When ready to serve, remove the congealed fat from the sauce, put the stew on the stovetop to warm, and follow the directions to complete the recipe.

When the venison is done, add the mushrooms and liquid accumulated with the mushrooms to the Dutch oven along with the green beans or peas. Continue cooking the stew for another 10 to 15 minutes. Remove the Dutch oven, uncover, and, working against the side of the pot, ladle the sauce into a saucepan and remove as much fat as possible (from the sauce). Bring the sauce to a boil, reducing it by half. Taste for seasoning, then pour the sauce over the venison and mix together again. To serve, garnish with the parsley.

Yield: 6 to 8 servings

Vinaigrette Salad

Cancer-fighting, calcium-containing crunch

Prep Time: 10 minutes
Cook Time: None

Ingredients

1 large head Bibb lettuce, washed and
chopped into bite-size pieces

1 ounce watercress, thoroughly washed
and tough stems removed

½ peeled carrot, sliced into long,
paper-thin strips with a vegetable
peeler

1 cup (150 g) grape tomatoes

1 tablespoon (15 ml) red wine vinegar

1 tablespoon (15 ml) freshly squeezed
lemon juice

1 tablespoon (15 ml) extra virgin
olive oil

¼ teaspoon Dijon mustard

¼ teaspoon raw honey

Sprinkling sliced almonds, optional

In a large serving bowl, combine the lettuce, watercress, carrot, and tomatoes.

In a small bowl, whisk the vinegar, lemon juice, oil, mustard, and honey. Pour over the salad. Toss to combine, sprinkle with the almonds, if using, and serve.

Yield: 6 servings

Notes from the Kitchen

- A quick cool salad, such as this simple Vinaigrette Salad made with basic ingredients, can be the perfect complement to a warming winter one-pot dish.

- You can use the zested lemon from the Venison Stew for the lemon juice in the Vinaigrette Salad.

Ingredients

2 teaspoons (10 ml) extra virgin
 olive oil

½ red onion, finely chopped

2 cloves garlic, minced

1 pound (455 g) leanest hamburger or
 ground turkey, optional

½ teaspoon liquid smoke

½ teaspoon salt

½ teaspoon ground black pepper

1 teaspoon dried oregano

3 cups (300 g) freshly cooked red beans
 or two 15-ounce (420-g) cans, rinsed
 and drained

1 red bell pepper, seeded and chopped

½ jalapeño pepper, seeded and finely
 chopped, or more to taste

1 large tomato, chopped, or one
 15-ounce (455-g) can diced tomatoes, drained (see "Notes from the
 Kitchen")

½ cup (120 ml) water

1 tablespoon (16 g) tomato paste

⅓ cup (33 g) Spanish olives, pitted and
 coarsely chopped

2 tablespoons (17 g) capers

2 cups (340 g) cooked long-grain
 brown rice

Red Beans, Brown Rice, and Lean Beef

Fiber and protein heavyweights

Prep Time: 15 minutes
Cook Time: 25 minutes

In a 4-quart (4-L) sauté pan, heat the oil over medium heat. Add the onion and garlic and sauté until translucent, about 5 minutes. Add the ground meat and cook until browned, about 5 to 6 minutes. Drain off any excess oil. Add the liquid smoke, salt, pepper, and oregano. Mix the spices into the meat and sauté for 2 minutes. Add the beans, bell pepper, jalapeño pepper, and tomato. Stir in the water and tomato paste. Bring to a simmer and cook for about 15 minutes. Stir in the olives and capers. Fold in the rice and serve.

Yield: 6 to 8 servings (about 10 cups [1700 g])

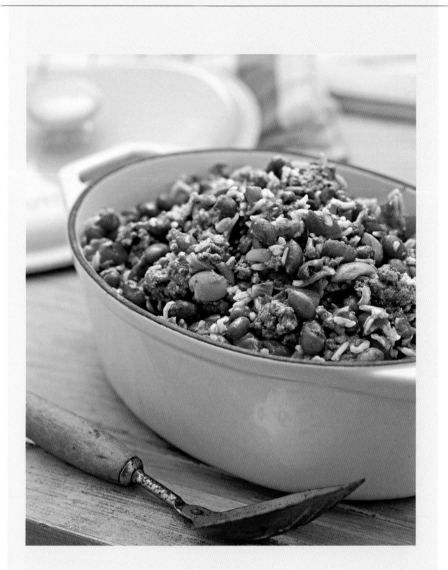

Notes from the Kitchen

- The theory of protein combining—the idea that you need to eat, for example, rice and beans together—is now largely discredited. As long as you get all the essential amino acids you need throughout the day, you don't need to eat them at the same time.

- The only thing missing in this dish is a little more green, so try it with steamed greens or green leafies with a sprinkling of nuts or seeds or a fresh green salad.

- This tasty dish works equally well with red meat, poultry, or as a vegetarian dish with neither!

- Traditional Cajun or Spanish red beans and rice dishes are usually cooked with some kind of ham hock and sausage or bacon. This dish gives you the same smoky flavor without all the poor-quality fat from a tiny amount of natural liquid hickory smoke. Also, the olives and capers give it a kicky flavor zing that more than replaces the richness of the lost meat oils.

- In place of the water and tomato paste, you could use half of the juice from the canned tomatoes or tomato juice.

Chapter 11 **Pantry List**

FOOD GROUP	FOOD	RECIPE
Dairy	Butter	Venison Stew
Grains	Long-grain brown rice	Red Beans, Brown Rice, and Lean Beef
	Whole wheat flour	Venison Stew
Herbs/Spices/Condiments	Bay Leaf	Venison Stew
	Black pepper (ground)	Lamb Chops and Sauerkraut; Red Beans, Brown Rice, and Lean Beef; Venison Stew
	Capers	Red Beans, Brown Rice, and Lean Beef
	Caraway seed	Lamb Chops and Sauerkraut
	Dijon mustard	Vinaigrette Salad
	Garlic	Red Beans, Brown Rice, and Lean Beef; Venison Stew
	Garlic powder	Lamb Chops and Sauerkraut
	Oregano (dried)	Red Beans, Brown Rice, and Lean Beef
	Parsley (fresh)	Venison Stew
	Salt	Lamb Chops and Sauerkraut; Red Beans, Brown Rice, and Lean Beef; Venison Stew
	Thyme	Lamb Chops and Sauerkraut, Venison Stew
	Worcestershire sauce	Venison Stew
Meat	Lamb chops	Lamb Chops and Sauerkraut
	Lean hamburger (or ground turkey)	Red Beans, Brown Rice, and Lean Beef
	Venison	Venison Stew
Miscellaneous	Broth (beef)	Venison Stew
	Broth (chicken)	Lamb Chops and Sauerkraut
	Liquid smoke	Red Beans, Brown Rice, and Lean Beef
	Olive oil (extra virgin)	Red Beans, Brown Rice, and Lean Beef; Venison Stew; Vinaigrette Salad

FOOD GROUP	FOOD	RECIPE
Miscellaneous	Raw honey	Vinaigrette Salad
	Red beans (fresh or canned)	Red Beans, Brown Rice, and Lean Beef
	Red wine vinegar	Vinaigrette Salad
	Sauerkraut	Lamb Chops and Sauerkraut
	White wine (dry)	Venison Stew
Nuts/Seeds	Almonds (or walnuts or pecans)	Steamed Green Veggies and Nuts, Vinaigrette Salad
	Almond oil	Lamb Chops and Sauerkraut
Produce	Apples	Lamb Chops and Sauerkraut
	Asparagus (or green beans or broccoli florets)	Steamed Green Veggies and Nuts
	Bibb lettuce	Vinaigrette Salad
	Carrots	Vinaigrette Salad
	Carrots (baby)	Venison Stew
	Crimini mushrooms	Venison Stew
	Grean beans, frozen (or baby peas)	Venison Stew
	Jalapeño pepper	Red Beans, Brown Rice, and Lean Beef
	Leeks	Lamb Chops and Sauerkraut
	Lemon juice	Vinaigrette Salad
	Lemon zest	Venison Stew
	Onions	Venison Stew
	Potatoes (red baby)	Venison Stew
	Red bell pepper	Red Beans, Brown Rice, and Lean Beef
	Red onion	Red Beans, Brown Rice, and Lean Beef
	Spanish olives	Red Beans, Brown Rice, and Lean Beef
	Tomatoes	Venison Stew; Red Beans, Brown Rice, and Lean Beef
	Tomatoes (grape)	Vinaigrette Salad
	Watercress	Vinaigrette Salad
	Tomato paste	Red Beans, Brown Rice, and Lean Beef

Clockwise from top left:
Simple Side: Spaghetti Squash,
Simple Side: Lemon-Herb Salad,
Schlemmertopf-Roasted Pesto
Chicken, Turkey Chili with Cashews
and Kale, Tangy Tomato Fish Stew,
Slow-Cooker Chicken Curry, Simple
Side: Plain Brown Rice, Simple Side:
Caesar Salad

CHAPTER 12

Poultry and Fish One-Pots

MEALS:

280 Schlemmertopf-Roasted Pesto Chicken

282 Simple Side: Lemon-Herb Salad

284 Turkey Chili with Cashews and Kale

286 Simple Side: Spaghetti Squash

288 Slow-Cooker Chicken Curry

290 Simple Side: Plain Brown Rice

292 Tangy Tomato Fish Stew

294 Simple Side: Caesar Salad

THE FOUR MEALS in this chapter all feature either poultry or fish, both of which are superb sources of protein, surrounded by a cornucopia of taste accents, superstar vegetables such as kale, and some combination of the "awesome foursome" of cooking ingredients: red wine, garlic, onions, and olive oil. But as the saying goes, "God is in the details," so let's get right to them.

A TASTY TRIO: GARLIC, RED WINE, AND OLIVE OIL

Our first meal, **Schlemmertopf-Roasted Pesto Chicken**, features an interesting triumvirate of supporting players: garlic, red wine, and olive oil. It's hard to see how you can go wrong with any meal featuring these three ingredients. Garlic, a member of the allium vegetable family, is the subject of well over 1,200 published studies. Its well-documented benefits include antimicrobial, antiviral, and antiparasitic activity, as well as some antihypertensive and antioxidant activity. What does all that mean in English? It means garlic helps kill bugs and bacteria, fights cellular damage, and may also lower blood pressure.

Garlic also lowers triglyceride levels by up to 17 percent. Why should you care? Simple. Triglycerides, the major form of fat in the human body that's also found in the bloodstream and is a component of all types of cholesterol, is an independent risk factor for heart disease. In the opinion of many—including me—triglycerides are far more of a risk factor and health concern than total cholesterol. Garlic can also reduce plaque, making it a double-duty weapon against cardiovascular disease.

If that weren't enough, compounds in garlic have been shown in a number of laboratory studies to be chemoprotective, meaning they help fight cancer. Research has demonstrated the ability of aged garlic extract to inhibit the proliferation of both leukemia cells and colorectal cancer cells. In areas where the consumption of garlic—and its allium vegetable family relatives—is high, there's a decreased risk of stomach and colon cancer. And garlic supplements also have a small but significant positive effect on blood pressure, modestly reducing it by 2 to 7 percent after 4 weeks of treatment.

Red wine is used in the Schlemmertopf-Roasted Pesto Chicken and also in the **Tangy Tomato Fish Stew**. You'll read more about it in Chapter 14, but let's just make mention of the fact that red wine is rich in a plant polyphenol called resveratrol, which is the subject of ongoing research for its antiaging properties. It's also a powerful antioxidant that offers certain health benefits in the prevention of heart disease and is known for its anticancer properties against a wide range of tumor cells. One group of resveratrol researchers, writing in the journal *Anticancer Research*, wrote that "resveratrol appears to exhibit therapeutic effects against cancer."

Olive oil is rich in monounsaturated fat, a "good" type of fat if there ever was one. (Except for hydrogenated oils—trans fats—and fats damaged by high heating such as deep frying, I'm not sure there's such a thing as a universally "bad" fat, but that's a whole other book. Nevertheless, even nutritionists who disagree over the "dangers" of fat are universally agreed that monounsaturated fat is "good.") Monounsaturated fat is found in high amounts in the famed Mediterranean diet, which is known to be associated with significantly reduced rates of heart disease. Besides in the Schlemmertopf-Roasted Pesto Chicken, olive oil is also found in the **Turkey Chili with Cashews and Kale** and in the Tangy Tomato Fish Stew.

KALE FOR WHAT AILS (YOU)

I'm not a big believer in ranking foods, because not even the greatest food in the world can provide everything the human body needs. (That's why I didn't assign rankings to top foods in my book *The 150 Healthiest Foods on Earth*.) But if pressed to name the top ten foods available, it would be hard not to include kale, the featured vegetable in the Turkey Chili with Cashews and Kale.

Kale consistently tests highest—or very close to highest—in the gold standard test of antioxidant power known as the ORAC test (oxygen radical absorbance capacity). That means that its particular combination of antioxidants—vitamins, minerals, and phytochemicals—performs together much like the Los Angeles Lakers in a championship season. They're an unbeatable team, and they are able to work together in a way that's more than the sum of their parts. In the bargain, they quell some of the nastiest and most dangerous of the free radicals, rogue molecules that cause cellular damage and are implicated in a wide range of diseases as well as the very process of aging itself.

Because it's a cabbage—and a member of that family of vegetable royalty known as the Brassica family—kale has even more benefits than its antioxidant power alone would indicate. It contains powerful phytochemicals known as indoles that have been found to have a protective effect against colon, cervical, and breast cancers. It's also high in a compound called sulforaphane, which helps give a boost to the body's detoxification enzymes. Sulforaphane triggers the liver to remove free radicals and other chemicals that may well cause DNA damage. In addition, kale contains calcium, iron, vitamins (A, C, and bone-building K), plus seven times the beta-carotene of broccoli. Kale also has almost ten times as much lutein and zeaxanthin, the new superstars of eye nutrition, as broccoli does. Lutein and zeaxanthin, which are both members of the carotenoid family that also includes beta-carotene, have been found to be very helpful in protecting against macular degeneration, the major cause of adult blindness.

Along with kale, you'll get plenty of onions, another superfood, in the chili. Onions and garlic, which I sang the praises of earlier, are kind of like kissing cousins. Both are members of the same allium vegetable family and share many of the same healthy properties. In a number of impressive studies, consumption of onions demonstrated protective effects against stomach cancer, and eating onions and its allium relatives (such as garlic, scallions, and leeks) has been shown to lower the risk for prostate and esophageal cancer. In fact, in Vidalia, Georgia—home of the Vidalia onion and a place where onions are widely consumed—the death rate from cancer of the stomach is fully 50 percent lower than the national mortality rate from stomach cancer.

And in a study published in the *European Journal of Clinical Nutrition*, onions were one of a very select group of foods that in combination was found to reduce coronary heart disease by an impressive 20 percent. (The others were broccoli, tea, and apples, which are all featured throughout this book.) Besides the Turkey Chili with Cashews and Kale, you'll also find onions in the **Slow-Cooker Chicken Curry** and Tangy Tomato Fish Stew.

CANCER-FIGHTING BROCCOLI

Also on that "hold a gun to my head and name the top ten foods" list is broccoli, which plays the "role" of kale as featured vegetable in the Slow-Cooker Chicken Curry.

Broccoli, like kale, is a member of the Brassica family, and also like kale, is simply loaded with antioxidants, vitamins, minerals, and other healing plant compounds. Chief among them are the indoles that, as mentioned above, have a protective effect against several types of cancer.

Broccoli is an excellent source of a whole family of anticancer phytochemicals called isothiocyanates, which fight cancer by neutralizing carcinogens—chemical agents known to be cancer promoting. Isothiocyanates do their good work by reducing the poisonous effects of the carcinogens, stimulating the release of carcinogen killers, and speeding up removal of carcinogens from the body. Studies have demonstrated that isothiocyanates help prevent both lung and esophageal cancers, can lower the risk of gastrointestinal cancer, and can inhibit tumors induced by chemical carcinogens. Broccoli in particular contains a potent isothiocyanate that inhibits mammary tumors. Researchers from Canada and the United States reported that an increased

Finishing Oils and Flavored Vinegars

They say variety is the spice of life, so here are some finishing oils you might want to try: white truffle oil, black truffle oil, hazelnut oil, sesame oil, almond oil, and macadamia oil. Experiment with different flavors and enjoy.

You can also be adventurous and make your own flavored vinegars as a way of adding some zip to your foods, especially vegetables and salads. Making flavored vinegars is safe, as it does not support the growth of *C. botulinum* bacteria due to its acid nature (as opposed to making your own flavored oils, which can pose a risk if not done properly). You can make some quite exotic-flavored vinegars such as dill, thyme, rosemary, raspberry, and strawberry.

intake of cruciferous vegetables was associated with a whopping 40 percent reduction in prostate cancer risk, and broccoli (and cauliflower) were singled out as offering the most protection.

And—this just in!—as we were going to press, a study in the *Journal of Neuroscience* suggested that broccoli may help the brain heal after an injury. A potent chemical called sulforaphane, which is found in broccoli and some other cruciferous vegetables, may help heal an important structure in the brain that acts primarily to protect it from harmful chemicals. This structure—a kind of membrane called the blood-brain barrier—is less efficient and effective after a brain injury. You can think of the blood-brain barrier as a kind of tightly woven "chain-link fence" keeping chemical riffraff out of the delicate tissues of the brain. But the fence starts to come apart after injury to the brain and loses some of its ability to act as an effective guard.

But researchers found that treating animals with sulforaphane helped lessen this effect, essentially helping to protect the brain from further damage and, in a real sense, helping it to heal from injury. If this promising research translates to humans it could add another feather in the cap of what is already one of the most nutritious and health-giving vegetables on the planet.

TURMERIC: SUPER SPICE

Another thing that makes these four dishes extraordinary is the cast of supporting characters: the spices. We really underestimate the medicinal properties of spices. Not only do spices—artfully used—make our foods taste amazing, but they are a rich (and often unrecognized) source of powerful phytochemicals with a wide range of healing and health-supporting properties.

The spice "star" of the Slow-Cooker Chicken Curry is turmeric. As in all curry dishes, turmeric is the spice that produces the characteristic yellow color. If ever there was a spice that deserved the label superfood, this yellow spice from India is it.

Turmeric contains many chemical compounds, but the family of compounds thought to be responsible for most of turmeric's considerable medicinal effects are the curcuminoids, the most important of which is called curcumin. Turmeric has phenomenal anti-inflammatory properties, and precisely for that reason, one of its many traditional uses has been for the treatment of arthritis. It's also one of the most "liver-friendly" spices, largely through its strong antioxidant activity. In science jargon, curcumin "inhibits lipid peroxidation." In English, that means it fights damage from oxidating substances that age the body and contribute to disease.

If that were all turmeric did, it would be impressive enough. But it's not. At least thirteen published studies indicate that the curcumin found in turmeric has an antitumor effect, meaning it reduced the number or the size of tumors, or lowered the percentage of animals that develop them. And in one study, curcumin inhibited the growth of human colon cancer cells. While I'm certainly not claiming that turmeric cures cancer, I believe there are an awful lot of reasons to make this your go-to spice as often as possible!

ONE OF MY FAVORITES: COCONUT

I don't want to leave this introduction without at least a passing nod to one of my absolute favorite ingredients, coconut, also featured in the Slow-Cooker Chicken Curry. Anyone who read *The 150 Healthiest Foods on Earth* knows that I am a huge fan of coconut in all its forms: extra virgin coconut oil, coconut meat, and coconut flakes. Classic studies of the coconut-eating people on the islands of Tokelau and Pukapuka done a few decades ago showed that despite eating a "high-fat" diet in which a large percentage of their daily calories came from coconut, the islanders were virtually free of artherosclerosis, heart disease, and colon cancer. (These studies were recently brought into the spotlight again in the superb book by my friend Gary Taubes called *Good Calories, Bad Calories*, which is a must-read for anyone interested in why the "wisdom" behind low-fat diets for health is quite simply wrong.)

Coconut contains a special kind of saturated fat called medium-chain triglycerides, MCTs for short. These fats are very easy to metabolize, and the body prefers to use them for energy rather than store them as fat around your hips. (At the time of the research study, the Pukapuka and

Tokelau islanders were supremely lean and healthy.) And 50 percent of the fat in coconut is lauric acid, which is a particular fatty acid that in the body morphs into an immune-boosting chemical called monolaurin. Monolaurin is basically a bug killer. It's antiviral and antibacterial, and its effects on a host of microbes demonstrate its immune-enhancing power. Another 6 to 7 percent of the fat in coconut is a fatty acid called capric acid, which morphs into monocaprin, a chemical shown to have antiviral effects as well. In short, coconut tastes great, and it supports your health in a myriad of ways, not the least of which is by enhancing immunity.

LEAN, MEAN PROTEIN

All four of these meals offer excellent protein. In our final recipe, Tangy Tomato Fish Stew, you'll enjoy halibut, which is a favorite of sushi eaters everywhere. Fish in general is a high-protein, low-calorie food that provides a range of health benefits. Four ounces of the typical whitefish contains approximately 27 g of protein. Halibut also has more potassium than a banana, and it offers some phosphorus and selenium as well. If you prefer, you can substitute another whitefish for the halibut, such as cod, which in case you're ever on Jeopardy! is one of the five most popular fish in the United States.

In comparison to the fish in the stew, four ounces of the meat of a roasted chicken, such as our Schlemmertopf-Roasted Pesto Chicken and Slow-Cooker Chicken Curry, provides about 30 g of protein. Four ounces of cooked ground turkey, the type that you'll be using in the Turkey Chili with Cashews and Kale, provides more than 22 g.

These four recipes really demonstrate how it's possible for truly healthy food to also be transcendentally delicious.

Enjoy!

A Good Egg

The Caesar Salad side dish contains a raw egg. You may have heard from some experts that raw eggs are unsafe to eat because of possible salmonella contamination. Personally, I don't agree. According to Joe Mercola, D.O., only 1 in about 70,000 eggs is contaminated with salmonella, and salmonella doesn't infect healthy chickens. Use organic, free-range eggs, and your chances of getting a contaminated one become somewhat similar to your chances of getting hit by a meteorite.

So if you ask me, free-range, organic eggs from happy chickens are extremely safe. I throw them in the blender in my protein smoothies all the time, almost daily. However, if you're still nervous, you can reduce your risk by simply poaching the egg for 2 minutes first: gently place it in a small saucepan of simmering water. Set a timer for 2 minutes and fish it out with a slotted spoon when the timer goes off. Run it under cold water briefly and crack it into your blender to make the dressing. Some of the white will have hardened a bit.

Any egg containing incompletely cooked white or yolk can still carry a slight risk, but truly, the chances of getting an infected egg from organically raised, free-range chickens is minuscule.

Ingredients

1 whole 3½- to 4-pound (1½- to 1¾-kg) baking chicken, organs removed, rinsed with neck skin and fat removed

2 cups (80 g) loosely packed fresh basil leaves, washed and patted dry

¼ cup (115 g) raw filberts

4 tablespoons (60 ml) extra virgin olive oil

¼ cup (60 ml) plus 1 tablespoon (15 ml) red wine, divided

1 small clove garlic

1 teaspoon salt

¾ teaspoon fresh ground black pepper, divided

2 cups (475 ml) low-sodium fat-free chicken broth

2 cloves garlic, crushed

1 to 2 teaspoons (2 to 4 g) organic Better Than Bouillon, chicken flavor, optional

1 teaspoon dried basil

¼ cup (15 g) sliced sun-dried tomatoes, chopped (see "Notes from the Kitchen")

4 carrots, peeled and cut on the bias into ½-inch (1-cm) sections

2 zucchini, sliced thickly on the bias into long sections about ¾ inch (2 cm) wide

1½ cups (150 g) heirloom-variety large green beans, stems removed

½ cup (95 g) wild rice

Schlemmertopf-Roasted Pesto Chicken
A cardiovascular helpmate

Prep Time: 15 minutes
Cook Time: 90 minutes

Put the Schlemmertopf lid into the sink and cover it with cold water until completely submerged. Let it soak for at least 15 minutes.

Meanwhile, in a food processor, puree the fresh basil, filberts, oil, 1 tablespoon (15 ml) of the wine, 1 clove garlic, salt, and ½ teaspoon of the pepper together in a food processor in short pulses. Stop frequently to scrape down sides, continuing to pulse until the mixture is still a little chunky, but evenly chopped. Set the pesto aside.

Pour the broth into the Schlemmertopf and whisk in remaining ¼ cup (60 ml) of wine, crushed garlic, bouillon, dried basil, and the remaining ¼ teaspoon of pepper. Add the tomatoes, carrots, zucchini, beans, and rice to the broth. Pat the chicken dry and place it on top of the vegetables. Put the pesto under the skin of the chicken breast and coat the entire outer surface of the chicken, plus inside both cavities. (It's okay if some pesto falls into the broth.) Cover the pot and put it on the lowest rack in the cold oven. Set the oven to 425°F (220°C, gas mark 7) and bake for 90 minutes. (If you have an electric stove, which often runs hotter than flame, the chicken may be done in 1 hour and 15 minutes.)

When the chicken is done, be careful removing the Schlemmertopf lid because the steam inside is very hot. Remove the chicken from the pot and set it on a large platter. Skim as much fat from the broth as you can, and remove the rice and vegetables with a slotted spoon. Place the rice and vegetables around the chicken on the platter or in a separate bowl.

Yield: 6 servings

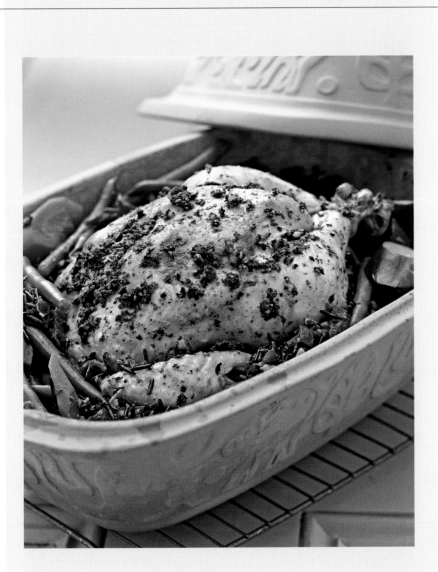

Notes from the Kitchen

- This dish is designed for the largest (turkey size) Schlemmertopf.

- A Schlemmertopf is a lidded terra-cotta pot. Although Schlemmertopfs aren't typical tools in American kitchens, they are staples in many European homes. Schlemmertopfs run a little pricey (around $70 for the larger models, less for used models sold online or secondhand), and they can be found in most good kitchen supply stores. They cook food so effectively and deliciously that they're worth the investment.

- To use your Schlemmertopf, soak the lid in cold water for about 15 minutes. While it is soaking, chop the vegetables. Assemble the ingredients, put them in the pot, and put on the wet lid. Place the pot on the low rack in a cold oven, then turn the oven temperature to 425°F (220°C, gas mark 7). Let your dish cook for between 60 and 90 minutes, depending on what you're making. (Whole chickens take longer; diced boneless cuts of meat take less time.) The wet lid will release moisture while your meal cooks. This combination of baking and steaming perfectly browns meat or vegetable skin, while cooking the insides to tender, juicy softness—perfect!

- Caution: Open the lid away from your face because the steam is very hot.

- The bouillon in the chicken dish is optional, but it does add a richer flavor.

- It's important to use dry sun-dried tomatoes for the chicken dish, not ones in oil. The dish is oily enough with the fat released from the chicken.

- Instead of zucchini, try quartered pattypans or golden yellow squash if they're in season.

Lemon-Herb Salad

A detox delight

Prep Time: 5 minutes
Cook Time: None

Ingredients

1 head chicory or escarole, cored,
   cut into bite-size pieces, well
   washed, and spun dry

1 to 2 tablespoons (15 to 28 ml)
   extra virgin olive oil

½ lemon

Dried oregano

Dried basil

Garlic powder

Place the chicory or escarole in a salad bowl. Drizzle the oil and squeeze the lemon over top. Generously sprinkle the oregano, basil, and garlic powder over the leaves, to taste. Toss well to combine.

Yield: 6 servings

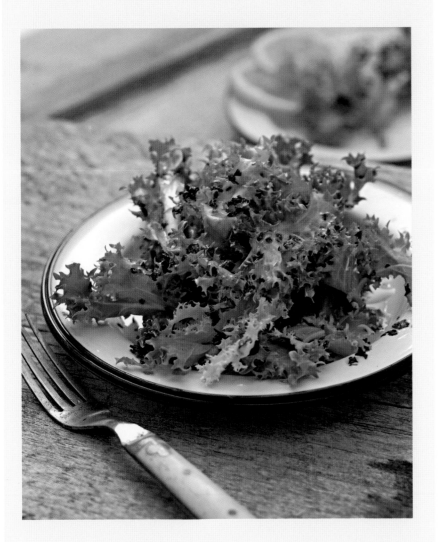

Notes from the Kitchen

- Escarole and chicory are related lettuce types. They are tougher, slightly more bitter options than the butterheads or romaine. Because they are somewhat toothier, they also do well steam-sautéed with garlic, seasonings, and nuts or seeds. Chopping the lettuce into bite-size pieces for a salad makes it easier to fork and chew. This Italian-style lemon and herb dressing is wonderful because it is so easy and you can make it as strong or mild as you wish.

- Don't be afraid to dress a quick salad right in the bowl. You can pair virtually any combination of oil and flavored vinegar (or in this case, citrus juice) that pleases your palate. Use equal parts oil and vinegar, about 2-3 tablespoons (28-56 ml) each, for a salad that serves 4-6 people. Then try sprinkling some savory herbs right onto the lettuce. The herbs in this salad will give it an Italian flavor, but you can try other combinations to give the same greens very different tastes. What about a sprinkling of tarragon and thyme for a hint of a French country garden?

Ingredients

1 tablespoon (15 ml) extra virgin
olive oil

1 yellow onion, finely diced

2 to 3 cloves garlic, minced

1½ pounds (680 g) ground turkey
or chicken

1 teaspoon dried oregano

2 tablespoons (15 g) chili powder

1 teaspoon ground cumin

¼ teaspoon ground cinnamon

½ teaspoon cayenne pepper

1 teaspoon salt

2½ cups (570 ml) low-sodium fat-free
chicken broth

1 cup (235 ml) dark beer

2 tablespoons (32 g) tomato paste

1 can (15.8 ounce, or 455 g) kidney
beans, drained

1 can (15.8 ounce, or 455 g) black
beans, drained

1 can (16 ounce 455 g) diced tomatoes
with mild green chilies

1 cup (150 g) colored bell pepper,
seeded and diced

1 small zucchini or yellow summer
squash, sliced into half rounds

1 cup (67 g) kale, stemmed and
chopped or torn into bite-size pieces

1 carrot, grated

¼ cup (31 g) cashews, chopped

½ cup (8 g) chopped fresh cilantro

1 to 2 tablespoons (15 to 28 ml) fresh
lime juice, optional

Turkey Chili with Cashews and Kale
A free-radical freedom fighter

Prep Time: 15 to 20 minutes
Cook Time: 30 to 40 minutes

In a 4- to 6-quart (4- to 6-L) sauté pan, heat the oil over medium heat. Add the onion and garlic and sauté until translucent, about 5 minutes. Add the turkey and cook until browned, for 5 to 6 minutes. Add the oregano, chili powder, cumin, cinnamon, cayenne pepper, and salt and sauté for 2 minutes. Pour in the broth and beer. Stir in the tomato paste. Add the kidney beans, black beans, tomatoes, bell pepper, zucchini or squash, kale, and carrot. Bring to a simmer, reduce the heat to low, cover, and cook for about 20 minutes, stirring occasionally. Add the cashews and cook for 5 to 7 minutes. Add the cilantro and lime juice, if using.

Yield: About 8 servings (about 12 cups [3 L], plus extra broth)

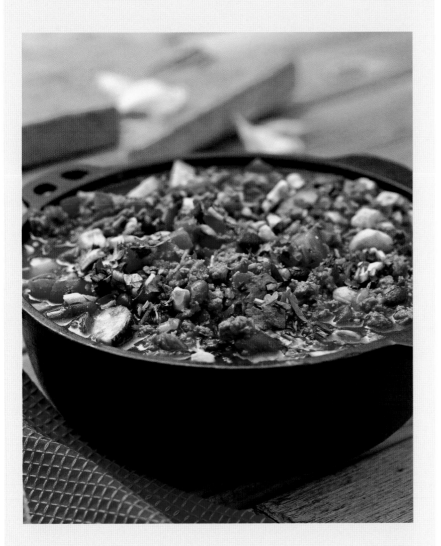

Notes from the Kitchen

- Traditionally, chili is cooked in large batches. If you aren't serving a crowd, plan to eat the leftovers throughout the week or store extras in the freezer: Let the chili cool for about 15 minutes and store it in a freezer-safe container in the refrigerator overnight. In the morning, remove the lid and dry all the condensed moisture with a paper towel. (This helps to reduce freezer burn.) Reseal the container, removing as much air as possible, and store it in your freezer for up to a month.

- There is no need for the excessive saturated fats of traditional chilis. You can make a very flavorful chili without even using meat. Keep beans as the primary ingredient. If you do use meat, choose a low-fat option, such as the ground turkey or chicken used in this recipe, to help reduce the calories of the dish. You could even make chili with ground buffalo.

- Chilis are very versatile, and you can use your own palate and intuition to customize any recipe. Add any combination of softer vegetables you happen to have in the fridge. If you want to use a slow cooker, just pre-brown and drain the meat, add all ingredients to the slow cooker, and cook for about 4 hours on high, or 8 on low.

- In this recipe, instead of the ground turkey or chicken, you can use about 3 cups (330 g) cubed or shredded cooked turkey or chicken. Add the cooked meat in with the tomatoes for the last 5 minutes of cooking time.

- If you like your chili hot, simply add more chili powder and/or cayenne pepper.

Spaghetti Squash

Low-cal faux pasta

Prep Time: 2 minutes
Cook Time: 1 hour, plus 20 to 30 minutes cooling time

Ingredients

1 small to medium spaghetti squash
  (4 to 6 pounds or 2 to 3 kg)
Seasonings, to taste (see "Notes from
  the Kitchen")

Preheat the oven to 375°F (190°C, gas mark 5).

Pierce the squash several times with a heavy pronged fork or sharp knife and place it in a baking pan. Bake for 1 hour, or until the flesh is tender when lightly pressed.

Remove the pan from the oven and let the squash cool for 20 to 30 minutes to avoid burning when you cut and seed it. Using oven mitts, cut the squash open lengthwise and scoop out the seeds with a spoon. Use a long fork to pull the strands free and place them in a bowl. Season the squash to taste.

Yield: 4 to 6 servings (about 5 to 7 cups [1125-1575 g])

Notes from the Kitchen

- Spaghetti squash, although a winter squash, has far fewer calories than its denser counterparts. One cup has only 42 calories! Choose a firm, heavy squash with even color and no dark spots. Squash keeps in a cool pantry for almost a month. The texture is watery in nature and the taste is very mild, so it does well with sharply flavored seasonings, or even a tangy tomato sauce.

- For faster preparation of the Spaghetti Squash, boil the whole squash. Place it in a very large pan of boiling water and cook for 20 to 30 minutes. It's ready when it pierces easily with a fork.

- To season the Spaghetti Squash, try a little salt, pepper, and butter; any combination of herbs or even a light vinaigrette. Or try a mixture of salt, butter, and Mexican spices such as chili powder and cumin to taste; even a touch of cayenne or dash of hot sauce will complement the chili and give it a kick.

Ingredients

1 teaspoon each salt, ground
black pepper, ground cumin, ground
coriander, and ground cardamom

½ teaspoon each ground cinnamon,
ground cloves, and ground turmeric

3 to 4 boneless skinless chicken thighs
(about 1 pound or 455 g)

4 boneless skinless chicken breasts
(about 2 pounds or 900 g)

1 large sweet onion, sliced and
separated into rings

3 medium carrots, sliced thin

2 large sweet potatoes, peeled
and cubed

1 can (8 ounce or 225 g) sliced water
chestnuts, drained

2 cups (475 ml) low-sodium fat-free
chicken broth

½ cup (120 ml) coconut milk

1½ tablespoons (9 g) curry powder

1 tablespoon (15 ml) fresh-squeezed
lemon juice

1 teaspoon salt

½ teaspoon crushed red-pepper flakes,
optional

2 tablespoons (12 g) finely chopped
fresh ginger

1 clove garlic, minced

2 cups (140 g) fresh broccoli florets, cut
into bite-size pieces

½ cup (115 g) plain low-fat yogurt

⅓ cup (6 g) chopped fresh cilantro,
optional

Slow-Cooker Chicken Curry
Cancer-fighting crudités

Prep Time: 1 hour for rub flavors to penetrate chicken plus 15 minutes
Cook Time: 4 to 5 hours on low or 3 hours on high

To make the spice rub: in a small bowl, combine the salt, pepper, cumin, coriander, cardamom, cinnamon, cloves, and turmeric. Set aside.

To make the chicken: Wash the chicken and pat to dry. Place the chicken in a large bowl. Sprinkle the spices over the chicken and use your hands to thoroughly coat it. Cover the bowl and place it in the refrigerator for 1 hour. Remove the chicken from the refrigerator.

Cover the bottom of the slow cooker with the onion. Sprinkle the carrots over the onions and top with the sweet potatoes and water chestnuts.

In a small bowl, whisk together the broth, coconut milk, curry powder, lemon juice, salt, red-pepper flakes, ginger, and garlic. Pour half of the broth mixture over the vegetables in the slow cooker. Place the chicken on top of the vegetables. Pour the rest of the broth mixture gently over the top.

Cook on high for 3 hours or low for 4 to 5 hours, or until the chicken is cooked through. Place the broccoli on the top for last 15 minutes of cooking time.

At the end of the cooking time, remove the chicken and place it in a large bowl. Skim the fat from the surface of the broth. Gently stir in the yogurt and cilantro if using. Pour the curry sauce over the chicken.

Yield: 6 servings

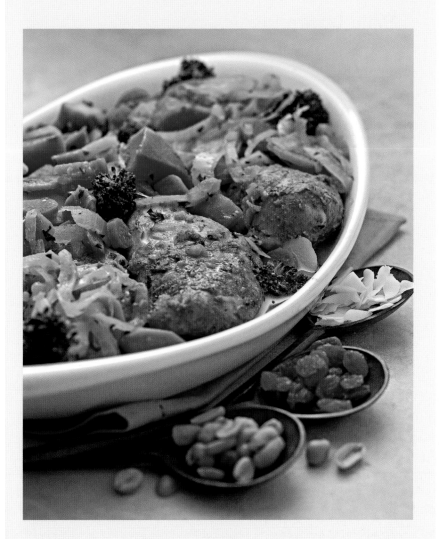

Notes from the Kitchen

- This curry is great served with bowls of shelled peanuts, raisins, and unsweetened dried coconut.

- To lower the fat content of the Slow-Cooker Chicken Curry, use all breast meat. Or you can use a 3- to 3½-pound (1¼- to 1½-kg) whole chicken, cut up into parts; however, reduce the broth content by ½ cup (120 ml).

- Slow cookers are a great for making one-pot meals because they are so easy to use. They are generally very inexpensive, ranging from $15 to $35, depending on the size. You can get them with high, low, and high-low settings. Some even have timers so they can be set to turn off on their own. Most hard grains and beans take a long time to cook in slow cookers and may even require some precooking, so they are best not included in dishes using proteins and more delicate vegetables. The best vegetables for slow-cooker stews are medium-soft ones (such as winter squash, potatoes, tomatoes, and onions) or hard ones cut very small (such as carrots sliced into thin rounds or finely diced rutabaga). Place onions and the hardest vegetables on the bottom of the pot. Then add the softer vegetables and top off with the meat. Pour the liquids over everything. There's no need for a lot of added liquids because there is very little evaporation in a slow cooker. Add broccoli and other quick-cooking green veggies for the last 15 minutes of cooking time.

- When making the spice rub, you can grind all these spices fresh for best flavor impact, or simply use powdered forms.

Plain Brown Rice

Fiber on the side

Prep Time: 3 to 5 minutes
Cook Time: 45 to 50 minutes, plus 5 to 10 minutes to rest

Ingredients

1 cup (190 g) brown basmati rice, medium grain brown rice, or long grain brown rice, rinsed and soaked (see "Notes from the Kitchen" on page 291)

2 cups (475 ml) water or no-sodium added broth

Pinch salt or splash of ume plum vinegar

Rinse the rice well and strain it through a colander or sieve.

In a pot with a tightly fitting lid, place the rice, water or broth, and salt or vinegar. Cover the pot. Cook over high heat until boiling, then reduce heat to low. Simmer for 45 to 50 minutes until the water is absorbed. Remove the pot from the heat and let rice sit for 5 to 10 minutes, then fluff it with a wooden spoon.

Yield: About 6 servings

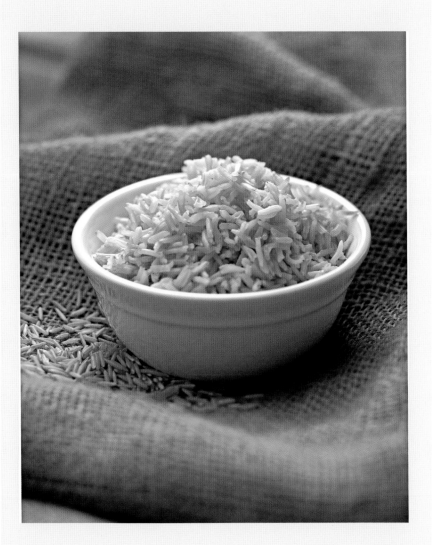

Notes from the Kitchen

- Long grain brown rice is a little drier and stays separate when cooked. Medium grain brown rice tends to stick together more. Medium and short grain rices have a slightly chewier texture than long. Basmati rice is the most aromatic of the three, with a wonderful, nutty smell when cooked.

- To make whole grains and beans more digestible and reduce the cooking time, rinse and soak them for 3 to 6 hours or overnight before cooking. (No need to do this with kasha, toasted buckwheat, or smaller grains such as quinoa and amaranth.) Be sure to throw off the soak water and start with fresh water in the cooking pot.

- If you have a hard time getting your rice—brown or other—perfect, consider one of the world's best inventions: the rice cooker. They are easy to use, keep rice warm until you're ready to enjoy it, and are virtually fail-proof. In general, all ingredients are combined using ¼ to ½ cup (60 to 120 ml) less liquid than the conventional stovetop method. Once you turn the cooker on, it will stop automatically when done because it senses a rise in temperature that occurs once all the liquid has been absorbed. There is no need to stir; in fact, stirring will release starches and cause the rice to become overly sticky. Make sure that the cooker you choose can also handle a wide variety of rices and whole grains, not just the traditional white rice. Once you start using a rice cooker, you'll realize its wonderful versatility in cooking anything from soups to stews, steamed meats, and vegetables.

Ingredients

3 tablespoons (45 ml) extra virgin olive oil

1 cup (100 g) thinly sliced celery (about 3 stalks)

1 red onion, chopped

3 cloves garlic, crushed and chopped

1 bulb fennel, cored, green tops removed and chopped

1 cup (82 g) tender baby or Italian eggplant (fits in palm of your hand, about 4 ounces), stem section removed and diced into ½-inch (1-cm) cubes, optional

1 cup (235 ml) full-bodied red wine

1 can (28 ounce, 784 g) or 2 cans (14.5 ounce, 420 g) diced tomatoes with juice

4 cups (946 ml) low-sodium fat-free chicken broth (1 carton [32 ounce, or 1 L carton])

½ teaspoon dried dill weed

1 teaspoon dried sweet ground fennel

¼ teaspoon cayenne pepper

2 dashes hot sauce or 1 dash habanera sauce

1 bay leaf

1 teaspoon salt

½ to 1 teaspoon ground black pepper

1 pound (455 g) wild halibut, skinned, any bones removed, and cut into 2-inch (5-cm) pieces

1 tablespoon (15 ml) fresh-squeezed lemon juice

Zest of ½ lemon

Tangy Tomato Fish Stew

A potful of potassium

Prep Time: 15 to 20 minutes
Cook Time: About 40 minutes

In a large soup pot, heat the oil over medium heat. Add the celery, onion, garlic, and fennel and sauté for 3 minutes. Add the eggplant if using and sauté the vegetables until they start to soften and the eggplant just begins to brown, about 3 to 4 minutes more. Add the wine and simmer for 8 to 9 minutes, until most of the wine is cooked off. Add the tomatoes, broth, dill, fennel, cayenne, hot sauce, bay leaf, salt, and pepper. Increase the heat to high and bring to a low boil. Reduce heat to low and simmer for 20 minutes. Add the fish, lemon juice, and zest and simmer for another 5 minutes, or until the fish is cooked through but still tender.

Yield: 4 to 6 servings

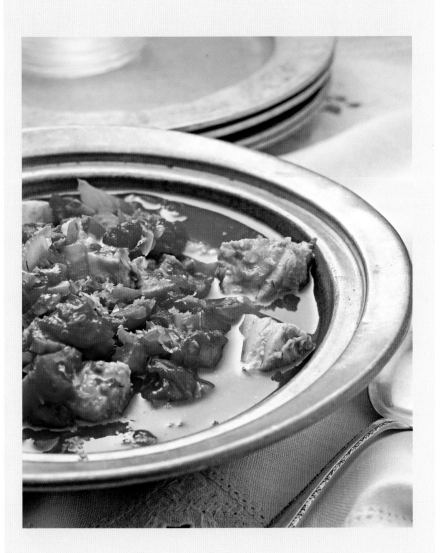

Notes from the Kitchen

- Fish stew is best made on the stovetop rather than in a slow cooker because the flesh is very tender and quick-cooking.

- Stew is a great way to get non-seafood fans to eat fish because stewing with a good flavor base and broth can remove a lot of the fishy taste that some folks find unpleasant.

- You can use haddock, pollock, or even thicker cod in place of the halibut. Cod will taste a little fishier, however.

- Try using heavy tweezers or needle-nosed pliers to debone raw fish.

- Eggplant, while not particularly nutritionally loaded, is filling, low fat, and low calorie. It adds a density to otherwise light dishes, allowing you to forgo other less healthy starchy options. Although eggplant comes in many varieties, they all taste fairly similar; always choose smaller and younger eggplants and try to use them immediately. The older they are, the tougher and more bitter they become. Small, young varieties are the most tender and don't even need to be peeled.

- Cut eggplant right before adding it to the stew, because the flesh will start to darken very quickly.

- For a zippier stew, omit the eggplant. You'll get a spicier flavor pop as opposed to the muskier flavor layers created by the eggplant.

- We tried this recipe using an inexpensive Cotes du Rhone and it was excellent.

Caesar Salad

A colon cancer warrior

Prep Time: 10 minutes
Cook Time: 2 minutes, if poaching the egg

Ingredients

1 tablespoon (16 g) anchovy paste

1 clove garlic, crushed

1 tablespoon (15 ml) lemon juice,
   freshly squeezed

1 raw or lightly poached egg

½ teaspoon Dijon mustard

Dash Worcestershire sauce

¼ cup (20 g) shaved Parmesan cheese,
   or to taste, plus more for topping

½ cup (120 ml) extra virgin olive oil

1 medium head romaine lettuce,
   washed and cut or torn into bite size
   pieces

In a blender or food processor, process together the anchovy paste, garlic, lemon juice, egg, mustard, Worcestershire sauce, and ¼ cup (20 g) of the cheese until well blended.

Place the lettuce in a large bowl. Add ¼ cup (60 ml) of the dressing, or more or to taste, toss well, and serve. Add additional grated Parmesan if desired. Refrigerate the unused dressing.

Yield: About 6 servings (plus extra dressing)

Notes from the Kitchen

- Leftover whole grains are great for other uses. Throw them into soups or salads to increase the fiber content or blend them with beans to make chewy veggie burgers. Sweeten them with a little juice or dried fruit, reheat, add a few nuts or seeds, and enjoy as a hot cereal.

- There's really nothing like the taste of fresh grated Parmesan. An easy way to get some variety in your dishes is to experiment with the many varieties of Parmesan cheese available at your grocer or local cheese store. Each has a slightly different characteristic; get to know them. With some creative experimentation—mixing specific dishes with the qualities of the various cheeses—you can seem like a gourmet chef. And when it comes to Parmesan cheese, a small amount can have big flavor!

Chapter 12 **Pantry List**

FOOD GROUP	FOOD	RECIPE
Dairy	Eggs	Caesar Salad
	Parmesan cheese	Caesar Salad
	Plain yogurt	Slow-Cooker Chicken Curry
Grains	Brown basmati rice (or other brown rice)	Plain Brown Rice
	Wild rice	Schlemmertopf-Roasted Pesto Chicken
Herbs/Spices/ Condiments	Basil (dried)	Schlemmertopf-Roasted Pesto Chicken, Lemon Herb Chicken
	Basil leaves (fresh)	Schlemmertopf-Roasted Pesto Chicken
	Bay leaf	Tangy Tomato Fish Stew
	Black pepper (ground)	Schlemmertopf-Roasted Pesto Chicken, Slow-Cooker Chicken Curry, Tangy Tomato Fish Stew
	Cardamom (ground)	Slow-Cooker Chicken Curry
	Cayenne pepper	Tangy Tomato Fish Stew, Turkey Chili with Cashews and Kale
	Chili powder	Turkey Chili with Cashews and Kale
	Cilantro (fresh)	Slow-Cooker Chicken Curry, Turkey Chili with Cashews and Kale
	Cinnamon (ground)	Slow-Cooker Chicken Curry, Turkey Chili with Cashews and Kale
	Cloves (ground)	Slow-Cooker Chicken Curry
	Coriander (ground)	Slow-Cooker Chicken Curry
	Cumin (ground)	Slow-Cooker Chicken Curry, Turkey Chili with Cashews and Kale
	Curry powder	Slow-Cooker Chicken Curry
	Dijon mustard	Caesar Salad
	Dill weed (dried)	Tangy Tomato Fish Stew
	Fennel (dried sweet ground)	Tangy Tomato Fish Stew
	Garlic	Caesar Salad, Schlemmertopf-Roasted Pesto Chicken, Slow-Cooker Chicken Curry, Tangy Tomato Fish Stew, Turkey Chili with Cashews and Kale

FOOD GROUP	FOOD	RECIPE
Herbs/Spices/ Condiments	Garlic powder	Lemon-Herb Salad
	Ginger (fresh)	Slow-Cooker Chicken Curry
	Hot sauce (or habanera)	Tangy Tomato Fish Stew
	Oregano (dried)	Lemon-Herb Salad, Turkey Chili with Cashews and Kale
	Red pepper flakes	Slow-Cooker Chicken Curry
	Salt	Plain Brown Rice, Schlemmertopf-Roasted Pesto Chicken, Slow-Cooker Chicken Curry, Tangy Tomato Fish Stew, Turkey Chili with Cashew and Kale
	Seasonings (to taste)	Spaghetti Squash
	Turmeric	Slow-Cooker Chicken Curry
	Ume plum vinegar	Plain Brown Rice
	Worcestershire sauce	Caesar Salad
Miscellaneous	Anchovy paste	Caesar Salad
	Better Than Bouillon, organic chicken	Schlemmertopf-Roasted Pesto Chicken
	Black Beans	Turkey Chili with Cashews and Kale
	Broth (chicken)	Schlemmertopf-Roasted Pesto Chicken, Slow-Cooker Chicken Curry, Tangy Tomato Fish Stew, Turkey Chili with Cashews and Kale
	Dark Beer	Turkey Chili with Cashews and Kale
	Kidney beans (drained)	Turkey Chili with Cashews and Kale
	Olive oil (extra virgin)	Caesar Salad, Lemon-Herb Salad, Schlemmertopf-Roasted Pesto Chicken, Slow-Cooker Chicken Curry, Tangy Tomato Fish Stew, Turkey Chili with Cashew and Kale
	Red wine	Schlemmertopf-Roasted Pesto Chicken, Tangy Tomato Fish Stew

(continued on page 298)

(continued from page 297)

FOOD GROUP	FOOD	RECIPE
Nuts/Seeds	Cashews	Turkey Chili with Cashews and Kale
	Coconut flakes	Slow-Cooker Chicken Curry
	Coconut milk	Slow-Cooker Chicken Curry
	Filberts	Schlemmertopf-Roasted Pesto Chicken
	Peanuts (dry roasted or cashews)	Slow-Cooker Chicken Curry
Poultry	Chicken (baking)	Schlemmertopf-Roasted Pesto Chicken
	Chicken (boneless skinless breasts)	Slow-Cooker Chicken Curry
	Chicken (boneless skinless thighs)	Slow-Cooker Chicken Curry
	Turkey (ground or chicken)	Turkey Chili with Cashews and Kale
Produce	Bell pepper (red, orange, or yellow)	Turkey Chili with Cashews and Kale
	Broccoli	Slow-Cooker Chicken Curry
	Carrots	Schlemmertopf-Roasted Pesto Chicken, Slow-Cooker Chicken Curry, Turkey Chili with Cashews and Kale
	Celery	Tangy Tomato Fish Stew
	Chicory (or escarole)	Lemon-Herb Salad
	Eggplant (baby or Italian)	Tangy Tomato Fish Stew
	Fennel	Tangy Tomato Fish Stew
	Green beans	Schlemmertopf-Roasted Pesto Chicken
	Kale	Turkey Chili with Cashews and Kale

FOOD GROUP	FOOD	RECIPE
Produce	Lemon (juice of)	Caesar Salad, Lemon-Herb Salad, Slow-Cooker Chicken Curry, Tangy Tomato Fish Stew
	Lemon zest	Tangy Tomato Fish Stew
	Lime (juice of)	Turkey Chili with Cashews and Kale
	Onion (red, sweet, yellow)	Slow-Cooker Chicken Curry, Tangy Tomato Fish Stew, Turkey Chili with Cashews and Kale
	Raisins (golden)	Slow-Cooker Chicken Curry
	Romaine lettuce	Caesar Salad
	Spaghetti squash	Spaghetti Squash
	Sun-dried tomatoes	Schlemmertopf-Roasted Pesto Chicken
	Sweet potatoes	Slow-Cooker Chicken Curry
	Tomatoes	Tangy Tomato Fish Stew
	Tomatoes, (diced, with mild green chilies or fire roasted)	Turkey Chili with Cashews and Kale
	Tomato paste	Turkey Chili with Cashews and Kale
	Water Chestnuts	Slow-Cooker Chicken Curry
	Zucchini (or summer squash)	Schlemmertopf-Roasted Pesto Chicken, Turkey Chili with Cashews and Kale
Seafood	Wild halibut	Tangy Tomato Fish Stew

Clockwise from top left:
Flax Pancakes with Fruit Compote; Seeded Rice; Miso Bean Soup; Quinoa Risotto with White Beans, Arugula, and Parmesan over Steamed Seasonal Greens

Vegetarian One-Pots

MEALS:

312 Flax Pancakes

314 Simle Side: Fruit Compote

315 Simple Side: Steamed Seasonal Greens

316 Quinoa Risotto with White Beans, Arugula, and Parmesan

318 Miso Bean Soup

320 Simple Side: Seeded Rice

THE DEBATE about whether or not vegetarianism is the ideal lifestyle is one in which feelings, beliefs, and emotions run high. People become vegetarians for a variety of reasons. Many think it's a healthier option. Many do it for ethical and moral concerns about animals or because of concerns about the planet in general.

The issue of vegetarianism as a way of life is far more complex and nuanced than most people realize. And it's far from settled. The arguments on both sides can be compelling and deserve a fair hearing, but this book—which is, after all, a fun book about great meals and the healing powers of foods—is not the place to catalogue the arguments on both sides of the fence (much as I'd like to). So let's just agree on one basic premise: Getting more vegetables in your diet is almost always a good thing.

These terrific vegetarian dishes are great for vegetarians and for meat eaters as well. In fact, even if you are a meat eater, the one-pot meals in this chapter offer a really interesting selection of alternatives to have once in a while (or more frequently). And if you are a vegetarian, you'll find much to love in these unique combinations. They may even give you some ideas of your own; feel free to expand the basic concepts and run with them. And if you come up with any great recipes, be sure to send them to us! Maybe we'll use them in the next edition.

NO FLACK FOR FLAX

I'm especially excited about the **Flax Pancakes** in meal number one. Virtually every one of the ingredients is a superfood, which is not surprising because the recipe was suggested by my good friend and master chef Dana Carpender, author of *500 Low-Carb Recipes*. And what makes it extra cool is that pancakes would be very unlikely to make the short list of "healthy foods" for most people. Not so with these nutritional gems.

Hardly a health book written in the past century doesn't sing the praises of flaxseeds and flaxseed oil. "Wherever flaxseed becomes a regular food item among the people, there will be better health," said Mahatma Ghandi. Flaxseed was actually one of the original medicines, used by the father of modern medicine himself, Hippocrates. It's a major plant source of the essential omega-3 fatty acid, alpha-linolenic acid, an important nutrient known for its anti-inflammatory properties. And the seeds, from which the flax meal is made, are a great source of lignans, which have a whole host of benefits. They help protect against cancer, particularly the cancers that are hormone sensitive, such as breast, uterine, and prostate cancers. (Lignans are thought to be one of the reasons vegetarian women seem to have lower rates of breast cancer.) And researchers have also found that lignans inhibit the growth of human prostate cancer cells in test tubes.

You can really up the ante on the nutritional benefits of flax by making your own flax meal. It's so easy. Just buy the actual flaxseeds and grind 'em up in a coffee grinder. You'll ensure freshness and potency that way, with minimum fuss and muss. (It's always best to grind them just prior to use—that way the oils don't have a chance to go rancid!) Flax promotes cardiovascular and colon health, can boost immunity, promotes healthy skin, and helps stabilize blood sugar. And 4 tablespoons (28 g) of flaxseed meal provide 6 g of protein and an amazing 8 g of fiber. Try getting that from the typical fare at your local pancake house!

The "gym mat" variety of pancake we're accustomed to in the United States is loaded with sugar and very heavy in simple carbs, which is a virtual prescription for a Sunday morning nap fest! By contrast, these pancakes, with their flax base and fruit topping, have so much protein and fiber that they will keep you both satisfied and energized all morning long.

Rounding out the ingredient list for the pancakes are two of my absolute favorite protein sources, both of which make my top ten list of superfoods: eggs and whey protein powder. Let's take them one at a time.

THE INCREDIBLE, EDIBLE EGG

Eggs are nature's most perfect food. On three of the four common scales used to rate protein quality, eggs consistently score highest, soundly beating milk, beef, whey, and soy. (On the fourth way of measuring protein, they're all rated the same with a perfect score.) But besides providing high-quality protein, eggs are also one of the best sources of a nutrient called choline, which is essential for cardiovascular and brain function. (And by the way, the choline is in the yolks!) Choline is an essential part of a related compound called phosphatidylcholine, without which both fat and cholesterol accumulate in the liver. Choline also forms a compound in the body called betaine, which in turn helps lower a dangerous inflammatory compound in the body called homocysteine. High homocysteine levels considerably increase your risk for heart disease, strokes, and Alzheimer's disease. On top of that, the nutritious yolk of the egg is loaded with two of the new superstar nutrients for eye health, lutein and zeaxanthin. Nature knew what it was doing when it put those nutrients in the yolk; they're much better absorbed with a little fat!

SAY YEA TO WHEY

Whey protein powder is my hands-down favorite kind of protein powder. The protein is of very high quality, and the whey protein boosts the body's stores of an important amino acid called glutathione. Glutathione is a master antioxidant: It mops up free radicals and is intimately involved in the detoxification of carcinogens. The white blood cells and the liver both use glutathione to detoxify poisons in the body. Unfortunately, it's difficult to absorb glutathione from the diet or from supplements; it needs to be manufactured in the body. And the best way to do this is by giving the body the amino acid building blocks from which glutathione is made. Whey protein powder is one of the richest sources of these building blocks.

Whey protein also contains natural ACE inhibitors, which are substances that lower blood pressure and improve cardiovascular health. And it also improves immune function. It's loaded with immune-supporting compounds called immunoglobulins that have important disease-fighting abilities. On top of that, it seems to be a great tool in the battle to control appetite naturally. The translation of this fifteenth-century Italian expression, "Chi vuol viver sano e lesto beve scotta e cena presto," says it all: "If you want to live a healthy and active life, drink whey and dine early."

KEEN QUINOA

Moving down the list, the **Quinoa Risotto with White Beans, Arugula, and Parmesan** is a special treat for a number of reasons, not the least of which is how rich and delicious it is. Quinoa, which was known by the Incas as the "mother of grains," is actually not a grain but a seed. But who cares? It looks like a grain, tastes like a grain, and cooks like a grain. But it's a grain with a major distinction: It's higher in protein than any common cereal grain. The nutritional quality of quinoa has even been compared to that of dried whole milk by the Food and Agricultural Organization of the United Nations.

Quinoa also beats out wheat, barley, and corn for its calcium, phosphorus, magnesium, potassium, copper, manganese, and zinc content. It's particularly high in iron, with ½ cup (88 g) of the stuff providing almost 8 mg, far more than any cereal grain, and just for good measure, the same serving contains an impressive 5 g of fiber. If you're a grain eater—or even if you're not—you couldn't do much better than quinoa.

BEANS, MUSHROOMS, AND MORE

In case you missed my earlier rant about fiber and beans, let me give you the recap: Fiber is great, and we need more of it. Our Paleolithic ancestors got at least 50 g a day, and all the major health organizations recommend that we take in anywhere between 25 and 38 g a day. Americans get about 10 on a good day! Beans are an almost unparalleled way to get fiber into the diet, plus they're low glycemic, meaning they raise blood sugar slightly and slowly, both very good things. They're the "ultimate" blood sugar regulator!

The Best Fermented Foods and Why You Should Eat Them

Fermented foods are high on my list of superfoods for their taste and, just as importantly, their health benefits. If you're new to the fermentation world, consider this an opportunity to add some new exotic foods to your repertoire that will pay dividends on health in terms of lower cholesterol, stronger digestive and immune systems, and protection from cancer.

Foods that are not fermented contain an ingredient called phytic acid, which can block the absorption of nutrients. Fermented products, on the other hand, will stop the effect of the phytic acid and increase the availability of isoflavones, a substance that has been shown to be heart disease and cancer protective.

Fermented soy foods are some good examples. Consider natto (which has been shown to dissolve blood clots), miso (rich in isoflavones that are cancer protective), tempeh, soy sauce, fermented tofu, and fermented soy milk. Anything else is processed and a lot less healthy.

And for what it's worth, analysis of food questionnaires in the famous Harvard research project called the Nurses' Health Study found a significant reduced frequency of breast cancer in women who consumed a higher intake of common beans or lentils. What's more, it didn't take all that much to produce the result. Eating beans or lentils only two (or more) times per week resulted in a very nice 24 percent reduced risk. A number of compounds in beans—for example, saponins, protease inhibitors, and diosgenin—appear to have the ability to either inhibit cancer cells or protect cells from the type of genetic damage that may lead to cancer. Good to know.

Shiitake mushrooms deserve a mention as well. It's a variety of mushroom that's deeply valued around the world for its medicinal effects. It contains enzymes and vitamins that are not normally found in plants, such as all eight essential amino acids and one of the essential fatty acids as well, linolenic acid. Shiitake mushrooms also contain a polysaccharide called beta 1,3 glucan that has potent immune-stimulating effects.

Finally there's olive oil, garlic, and onions, all super performers that have been discussed at length throughout this book. If ingredients were rock stars, this trio would be the equivalent of the reunion of Cream. Olive oil is loaded with the healthy monounsaturated fat that's such an important part of the Mediterranean diet. Onions and garlic have both been associated with reduced risk of cancer, lowered blood pressure, and a reduced risk of heart disease. What's not to love about this dish?

MISO FOR YOU

Finally let's talk about the **Miso Bean Soup**, which is fast becoming a staple in the Bowden household for a number of reasons, not the least of which is how easy it is to prepare and how well it keeps in the fridge. Suggested by my friend Linda Page, this clever recipe combines some of our old friends and familiar ingredients such as eggs (see page 304), beans (see page 305), and onions (see page 306), but the predominant flavor and special ingredient is miso.

Miso is a soybean paste that's been a mainstay of Japanese cooking since the seventh century. It's made by mixing cooked soybeans with salt, a grain, and a fermenting agent called koji. A quarter cup (60 g) of miso contains about 8 g of soy protein as well as a respectable 3.7 g of fiber.

You can buy many varieties of miso. For example, hacho miso is made strictly from soybeans, and natto miso is made from ginger and soybeans. Most of the others are made from soybeans and a grain, such as white or brown rice, barley, or buckwheat. Mugi miso, which is made with barley, is the sweetest variety and great for soups and general cooking.

Traditionally fermented miso, like all traditionally fermented foods (such as yogurt, sauerkraut, and olives) is a rich source of healthy bacteria that can help balance your digestive system and increase the possibility that you will absorb and use all of the nutrients you eat.

The side dish that accompanies the Miso Bean Soup features pumpkin seeds, which are a rich source of minerals, especially magnesium, potassium, and phosphorus. Interestingly, roasted pumpkin seeds have more protein as well as more of the above-mentioned three minerals. They also have more zinc, fiber, and selenium. And both dry and roasted pumpkin seeds have a nice amount of manganese, which is an important trace mineral that's essential for growth, reproduction, wound healing, peak brain function, and the proper metabolism of sugars, insulin, and cholesterol.

Now if you'll excuse me, I'm going to go and make the pancakes!

Other fermented foods are good as well. Unsweetened yogurt is wonderful for digestion as the beneficial bacteria grows during the fermentation process. You can't go wrong with olives, with all the countless health benefits associated with them, including a lowered incidence of heart disease and certain cancers. Sauerkraut is another good choice. It's known by the Koreans as kimchee, and it is also very healing for the digestive tract.

But beware of commercially produced sauerkraut and pickles, which do not offer the same benefits. They are chemically treated, packed in salt, and canned. To avoid finding your health in a pickle later on, avoid the processed stuff and stick to fresh and healthy fermented choices. Asian markets are a great place to start.

The Importance of an Acid-Alkaline Balance

Here's another reason to eat your vegetables: They will help to balance your pH level, which in turn will help to prevent a myriad of diseases. The body likes to maintain blood pH of between 7.35 and 7.45. Anything lower than this range is considered acidic, and anything above this range is considered alkaline. When the body is too acidic, it has a hard time functioning properly and may be less efficient at absorbing nutrients, generating energy, repairing damaged cells, and detoxifying heavy metals. As a result, certain disease states can develop, including cancer.

You can test your urine pH with test strips that can be purchased at any pharmacy. Unlike blood, the urine pH reading should be between 5.8 and 6.8.

Foods are classified as either alkaline or acidic. Most Americans eat an acidic diet, high in meats, salts, and dairy. Fruits and vegetables, on the other hand, are very alkalizing. Use the guide below to help you achieve a healthy balance.

	ALKALIZING FOODS	ACIDIFYING FOODS
Fruits	Dates, figs, melons, grapes, papaya, kiwifruit, lemons, watermelon, limes, grapefruit, mangoes, apples, pears, raisins, avocados	Sour cherries, rhubarb, blackberries, cranberries, prunes
Vegetables, beans, and legumes	Asparagus, onions, vegetable juices, parsley, raw spinach, broccoli, garlic, green beans, beets, celery, lettuce, zucchini, sweet potato, carob	Potatoes, pinto beans, navy beans, lima beans, chocolate
Nuts and seeds	Almonds, chestnuts	Pecans, cashews, peanuts, walnuts
Grains	Amaranth, millet, wild rice, quinoa	Sprouted wheat bread, spelt, brown rice, white rice, corn, oats, buckwheat, rye, white flour, pastries, pasta
Meats	None	Beef, pork, shellfish, turkey, chicken, lamb
Eggs and dairy	None	Cheese, homogenized milk, ice cream, cottage cheese, yogurt
Beverages	Herb teas, lemon water, green tea	Beer, soft drinks, coffee, black tea

Flax Pancakes

You'll flip over these fatty acids and fiber

Prep Time: 5 minutes
Cook Time: About 3 minutes per batch

Ingredients

1 cup (115 g) flaxseed meal

1 cup (128 g) vanilla whey protein powder

¾ teaspoon baking soda

1 packet stevia

½ teaspoon salt

¼ cup (28 g) oat flour

1 teaspoon ground cinnamon

1 teaspoon macadamia nut oil or coconut oil, optional

1 cup (230 g) plain yogurt

2 eggs

In a mixing bowl, combine the flaxseed meal, protein powder, baking soda, stevia, salt, flour, and cinnamon and stir well to combine.

In a large skillet or griddle, pour the oil and set it over medium-high heat. (If your skillet or griddle has a good nonstick surface, you can skip the oil.)

While the oil heats, whisk the yogurt and eggs into the flaxseed mixture, making sure there are no dry pockets left.

When your skillet is hot enough that a drop of water will skitter across the surface, pour or wipe the excess oil out of the pan. (Be careful not to burn yourself!)

Scoop the batter with a ¼-cup (60-ml) measure into the pan. Cook the first side until bubbles start to show in the batter and the bottom edges begin to dry, about 1 minute. Then carefully flip the pancakes and cook the other side for 30 seconds to 1 minute, until they are cooked through but not too brown.

Serve with fruit compote or the topping of your choice.

Yield: 4 to 6 servings (12 to 14 small pancakes)

Notes from the Kitchen

- Optional toppings: fruit compote (see recipe, page 314), yogurt and honey, or crushed nuts/seeds, juice-sweetened jam, agave nectar, etc.

- The Flax Pancakes freeze beautifully. Let them cool to room temperature. Lay them side by side on a long piece of wax paper. Fold the pancakes and paper over and add another layer of pancakes until they are three pancakes thick. Place the wrapped pancakes into freezer-safe resealable plastic bags and remove the air. Rewarm the pancakes in the toaster oven when ready to eat. Don't refrigerate pancakes before freezing or they will get too chewy.

- Invest in an inexpensive coffee grinder, even if you already have one. Use the second one just for spices and flaxseeds. That'll keep your spices and flax from having a coffee flavor. Plus if you have a dedicated spice and flax grinder, you'll tend to use it more often!

- With all oils and with flaxseeds as well, quality and freshness are very important. For this reason, I recommend Barlean's for both flax products and coconut oil. It's a small, dedicated family company that markets only the highest-quality, organic flax and coconut oil, neither of which is expensive, and both of which are readily available in stores.

Fruit Compote

Berries feed a robust memory

Prep Time: 5 minutes
Cook Time: 10-15 minutes

Ingredients

2 cups (220 g) mixed berries or other
soft fruit, such as peaches or pears

2 to 3 tablespoons (28 to 45 ml) juice,
such as apple cider, orange, cherry,
or pomegranate

1 to 2 teaspoons agave nectar or raw
honey, optional

½ teaspoon sweet spices, such as
ground cinnamon, ginger, cardamom,
allspice, or nutmeg

2 teaspoons (5 g) kudzu

2 teaspoons (10 ml) cold water

½ teaspoon vanilla extract

Ground nuts, optional

In a medium saucepan, combine the fruit, juice, agave or honey if using, and spices. Heat on medium-high until it simmers. Reduce the heat to low and cover, watching carefully so it doesn't boil over. Cook the fruit down for 8 to 12 minutes, adding more juice, if necessary.

In a small bowl, mix the kudzu and water and pour into the saucepan. Stir for 20 to 30 seconds, until the compote thickens. Remove the saucepan from the heat, add the vanilla, and stir it in. Serve hot over pancakes. Sprinkle with the nuts if using.

Yield: 4 to 6 generous servings

Steamed Seasonal Greens

Great grains, protein, iron, and fiber

Prep Time: 5 minutes
Cook Time: 4 to 10 minutes

Ingredients

2 pounds (900 g) any tender greens, such as spinach, bok choy, escarole, or Swiss chard

½ to ¾ cup (120 to 175 ml) water or broth (can also add a splash of wine)

½ teaspoon salt

¼ teaspoon ground black pepper

Wash, stem, and coarsely chop the greens. Place them in a 4- or 6-quart (4- or 6-L) sauté pan and pour in the water or broth and wine, if using. Cover and cook on high until the liquid is at a high simmer. Add the salt and pepper and steam for 2 to 6 minutes until the leaves are well wilted and their green color deepens. (Delicate greens like spinach will cook faster; hardier greens like chard will take longer.)

Yield: About 4 servings

Notes from the Kitchen

• Here's a simple little rule for properly steaming greens, whether it be collards, bok choy, spinach, or any other fresh leafy green: Watch their color! When the color intensifies, they're done. Usually this takes about a minute or two (three, tops) for delicate greens, longer for hardier greens like collards or kale. This will maintain the texture as well as most of their nutrients. Easy, huh?

Spice Up Your Vegetables

Feel free to experiment with different herbs and spices on vegetables. The tried and true favorites are basil, chervil, chives, cumin, fennel, fines herbes, ginger, marjoram, paprika, parsley, savory, sesame seeds, and tarragon. Depending on the vegetable you can also use dill, rosemary, thyme, and coriander. The trick is to not overwhelm the vegetables with the herbs. Let the natural flavor still shine through; when you can, add herbs and spices a little at a time until the right balance is achieved.

Quinoa Risotto with White Beans, Arugula, and Parmesan

A nutritional powerhouse in tender form

Prep Time: 5 to 10 minutes
Cook Time: 15-20 minutes

Ingredients

1 tablespoon (15 ml) extra virgin
  olive oil

½ sweet yellow onion, chopped

1 clove garlic, minced

1 cup (175 g) quinoa, well rinsed

3 cups (705 ml) low-sodium
  vegetable broth

¼ to ⅓ cup (35 to 45 g) pine nuts

1 can (15.8 ounce or 455 g) organic
  great northern beans, drained and
  rinsed, or 2 cups (200 g) fresh-cooked
  beans

1 cup (70 g) thinly sliced fresh shiitake
  mushrooms

1 carrot, finely grated

2½ cups (50 g) rocket arugula,
  stemmed and chopped

¼ cup (25 g) fresh grated Parmesan
  cheese

½ teaspoon salt

¼ teaspoon freshly ground black
  pepper

In a large saucepan, heat the oil over medium heat. Add the onion and sauté until soft and translucent, about 4 minutes. Add the garlic and quinoa and cook for about 1 minute, stirring occasionally. (Don't let the garlic brown.) Add the broth, increase the heat to high, and bring to a boil. Reduce the heat to low and simmer until the quinoa is almost tender to the bite but slightly hard in the center, about 12 minutes. (The mixture will be brothy.)

While the mixture is cooking, toast the pine nuts in a dry frying pan over medium heat until they release their oils and fragrance, 3 to 4 minutes. (Do not overcook; browning makes them bitter.)

At 12 minutes (on the quinoa), stir in the beans, mushrooms, carrot, and arugula and simmer (increasing heat if necessary) until the quinoa grains have turned from white to translucent and their "tails" have popped, about 2 to 3 minutes longer. Stir in the cheese, season with salt and pepper, and sprinkle pine nuts over the top. Serve immediately.

Yield: About 4 servings

Notes from the Kitchen

- If you want to add a little more bite to the Quinoa Risotto with White Beans, Arugula, and Parmesan, try adding a sprinkle of Minus 8 or high-quality balsamic vinegar to finish the cooked dish.

- Try using red heirloom quinoa for a pretty dish.

- You can use fat-free chicken broth instead of vegetable broth in the quinoa, if you're not concerned about keeping it vegetarian.

- Don't limit your quinoa experience to just the delicious Quinoa Risotto with White Beans, Arugula, and Parmesan. Experiment. Quinoa cooks up just like oatmeal, and it makes a great substitute for a more traditional hot cereal. You can even mix it with oatmeal for an unusual "half and half." A number of cold cereals are now available that are based on quinoa.

- Quinoa makes a great substitute for a starchy side dish. It's great with a little organic butter and sea salt!

- This mild quinoa dish does well served simply over a bed of large-leaf lettuce. Or you can steam some seasonal greens briefly in a steamer basket as a side. Try it with whole baby bok choy in the late spring or young collards, stemmed and cut into ribbons, in the early fall.

Miso Bean Soup

Helps nutrient absorption

Prep Time: 5 minutes, plus soak time overnight
Cook Time: 90 minutes to 2 hours

Ingredients

1 pound (455 g) dried black beans
(2½ cups)

2 tablespoons (25 ml) extra virgin
olive oil

1 red onion, finely diced

2 cloves garlic, minced

8 cups (2 L) low-sodium
vegetable broth (2 cartons [32-ounce
or 1-L])

2 cups (475 ml) dry red wine, such as
Merlot

2 tablespoons (32 g) dark miso paste

1 teaspoon coarsely ground black
pepper

¼ cup (60 ml) port or Marsala wine

1 hard-boiled egg, crumbled, optional

Lemon slices, optional

Place the beans in a large bowl and cover them with water. Soak them overnight.

Rinse and drain the beans.

In a large pot, heat the oil over medium heat. Add the onion and sauté for 5 minutes. Add the garlic and sauté for 2 to 3 more minutes. Add the broth, red wine, and beans. Increase the heat to high and bring to a boil. Reduce the heat to low and simmer, partially covered, for about 2 hours, stirring occasionally. Add additional broth if necessary to keep beans covered with liquid. When the beans are cooked (tender to the squeeze, but still retaining their skins), remove the pot from the heat and stir in the miso. Puree the soup with a soup wand to the desired consistency. (If you don't have a soup wand, cool the soup slightly and puree it in batches in the blender and return to the pot.) Add the pepper and port or Marsala wine and stir to combine. Ladle the soup into shallow bowls and top with the egg and lemon, if using.

Yield: 6 to 8 servings

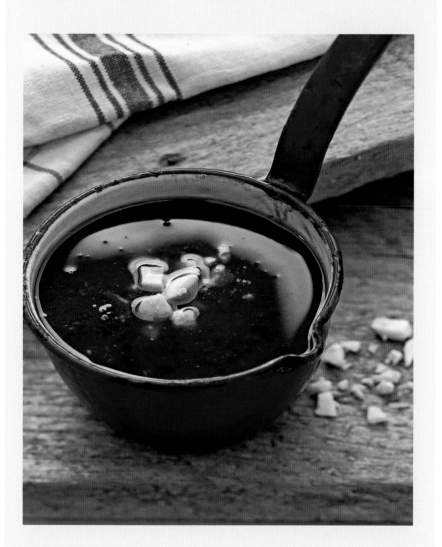

Notes from the Kitchen

- A simple bowl of soup makes a lovely cold-weather meal. Try it alone for a light lunch or snack or pair it with the seeded rice to beef up your protein, fiber, and essential fatty acids.

- Soup makes a great breakfast, especially if you're trying to lose fat in a healthy way. For simple soups at any time (even for breakfast), just simmer 1 cup (120-200g) of any veggies until soft and add 1 tablespoon (16 g) miso paste per 1½ cups (355 ml) liquid once removed from heat.

- You can buy a wide range of colors of miso, from white to brown. In a nutshell, the darker the color, the stronger, more intense, and saltier the flavor.

- Look for organic, unpasteurized miso with no chemicals or other additives. The commercial pasteurization destroys miso's wonderful beneficial bacteria and enzymes.

- Be careful when heating up your miso soup. Bring it to a simmer, but do not allow it to heat up past its boiling point, because that may decrease some of its great nutritional properties.

- To add veggies to this meal, a crudités platter, steamed greens, or a green salad would make great additions. (See Steamed Seasonal Greens on page 315 or Vinaigrette Salad on page 262.)

Seeded Rice

Pumpkin seeds for prostate health

Prep Time: 5 minutes, plus overnight if presoaking
Cook Time: 45 to 50 minutes, plus 5 to 10 minutes rest time

Ingredients

1 cup (190 g) whole grain rice, any variety

¼ cup (35 g) raw pumpkin seeds, sunflower seeds, or a combination

2¼ cups (535 ml) water or low-sodium vegetable broth

½ teaspoon ume plum vinegar or salt

Rinse the rice and drain in a colander or sieve. Place the rice in a large bowl and cover it with water. Soak the rice overnight.

Throw off the soaking water.

In a pot with a tightly fitting lid, combine the rice, seeds, water or broth, and vinegar or salt. Cook over high heat until boiling. Reduce the heat to low and simmer for 45 to 50 minutes. Remove the pot from the heat and let the rice sit for 5 to 10 minutes, then fluff it with a wooden spoon.

Yield: About 6 servings

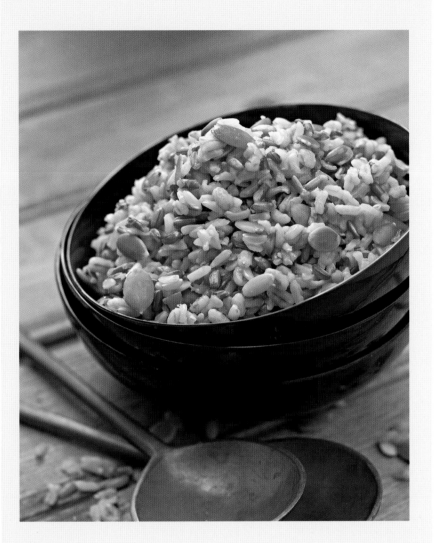

Notes from the Kitchen

- When making the Seeded Rice, try sweet brown rice for a stickier, chewier texture.

- You can be a little adventurous with the Seeded Rice by adding nuts, seeds, other grains, or even dried fruits to your cooked rices. The basic rule of thumb is that at least three-quarters of your mixture should be a whole grain rice; the final one-quarter can be a combination of different things. You may also need ¼ to ½ cup (60 to 120 ml) more liquid. Try pecans and cranberries, sunflower seeds and dried apricots, wheat berries, or pearled barley.

- For a side dish higher in nutrients, you can substitute quinoa for the rice. Remember that quinoa only needs about 15 minutes to cook, however, so you wouldn't want to use a rice cooker. Rinse it well (no need for presoaking), then follow the directions at left, but use 2 cups (475 ml) of liquid instead of 2¼ (535 ml) and cook for 15 to 20 minutes until translucent and the "tails" have popped.

- A wonderful Japanese barley called Hato Mugi or Job's Tears is great cooked with brown rice. You can buy it in most Asian grocers. It yields a fatter, chewier grain than traditional barley. A good rice cooker will take the guesswork out of the cooking time. Just throw it all in together, push the button, and voilà: great grains!

Chapter 13 **Pantry List**

FOOD GROUP	FOOD	RECIPE
Dairy	Eggs	Flax Pancakes, Miso Bean Soup
	Parmesan cheese	Quinoa Risotto with White Beans, Arugula, and Parmesan
	Plain yogurt	Flax Pancakes
Grains	Flaxseed meal	Flax Pancakes
	Oat flour	Flax Pancakes
	Quinoa	Quinoa Risotto with White Beans, Arugula, and Parmesan
	Whole grain rice	Seeded Rice
Herbs/Spices/Condiments	Black pepper (ground)	Miso Bean Soup; Quinoa Risotto with White Beans, Arugula, and Parmesan; Steamed Seasonal Greens
	Cinnamon (ground)	Flax Pancakes
	Garlic	Miso Bean Soup; Quinoa Risotto with White Beans, Arugula, and Parmesan
	Salt	Flax Pancakes; Quinoa Risotto with White Beans, Arugula, and Parmesan; Steamed Seasonal Greens
	Sweet spices (ground cinnamon, ginger, cardamon, allspice, or nutmeg)	Fruit Compote
	Vanilla extract	Fruit Compote
Miscellaneous	Agave nectar (or raw honey)	Fruit Compote
	Baking soda	Flax Pancakes
	Black beans	Miso Bean Soup
	Broth (vegetable)	Miso Bean Soup; Quinoa Risotto with White Beans, Arugula, and Parmesan; Seeded Rice
	Dark miso paste	Miso Bean Soup
	Great northern beans	Quinoa Risotto with White Beans, Arugula, and Parmesan
	Kudzu	Fruit Compote
	Olive oil (extra virgin)	Miso Bean Soup; Quinoa Risotto with White Beans, Arugula, and Parmesan
	Port wine (or Marsala)	Miso Bean Soup

FOOD GROUP	FOOD	RECIPE
Miscellaneous	Red wine (dry)	Miso Bean Soup
	Stevia	Flax Pancakes
	Ume plum vinegar (or salt)	Seeded Rice
	Vanilla whey protein powder	Flax Pancakes
Nuts/Seeds	Ground nuts	Fruit Compote
	Macadamia nut oil (or coconut oil)	Flax Pancakes
	Pine nuts	Quinoa Risotto with White Beans, Arugula, and Parmesan
	Pumpkin seeds (or sunflower)	Seeded Rice
Produce	Apple Cider (or orange, cherry, or pomegranate juice)	Fruit Compote
	Berries (mixed)	Fruit Compote
	Carrots	Quinoa Risotto with White Beans, Arugula, and Parmesan
	Greens (spinach, bok choy, escarole, or Swiss chard)	Steamed Seasonal Greens
	Lemon	Miso Bean Soup
	Onion (red)	Miso Bean Soup
	Onion (yellow)	Quinoa Risotto with White Beans, Arugula, and Parmesan
	Rocket arugula	Quinoa Risotto with White Beans, Arugula, and Parmesan
	Shiitake mushrooms	Quinoa Risotto with White Beans, Arugula, and Parmesan

Delicious Drinks:
The Liquid Polymeal

3

Clockwise from top left:
Sultry Summer Sangria,
Hunger Buster, Frozen Tropical Treat,
Antioxidants on the Run, Melon
Snap, Nut Power, Liver Support: The
Alkalizer, Sweet Morning Eye Opener

Beverages

DRINKS:

336 Sultry Summer Sangria

338 Liver Support: The Alkalizer

338 Jonny's Recipe for Supermarket SuperJuice

339 Liquid Polymeal Formula

340 Hunger Buster

340 Sweet Morning Eye Opener

342 Frozen Tropical Treat

344 Melon Snap

344 Nut Power

346 Antioxidants on the Run

REMEMBER the old saying "bread is the staff of life"? Guess what: It's a fairy tale. It sounded good, and was comforting to believe, but in the long run it's no more accurate than the idea of Santa Claus. Water, on the other hand, is a different story.

While it may not sound as romantic and biblical to say "water is the staff of life," it's actually true. You can live a lot of days without food. (Don't ask me how many. Hunger strikes have gone on for at least thirty, or you could ask the cast of the latest edition of Survivor.) But water? No way, José. Seven days max, and for the last two you'd be crazy. Water is needed for every metabolic process in the body. It flushes out toxins, is the medium in which cellular exchange of nutrients and other chemicals takes place, and is a large component of blood, tissue, muscle, and organs. It's utterly essential for life and arguably the best overall drink in the world.

So why drink anything else?

Well, actually, that's not an unreasonable question. Some answers that come quickly to mind: taste, pleasure, and variety; nutrients and phyto-chemicals; and of course, energy (i.e., calories). Shall I go on?

The problem, like so many things in life, is one of balance.

From a health point of view, the beverage world is a land mine. Since the introduction of high-fructose corn syrup in 1978, consumption of sugars has gone up in America exponentially, as has obesity. Much of this is fueled by beverage consumption. There's good evidence that drinking calo-ries is processed differently by the brain than eating them, and it's certainly pretty easy to down a supersize soda of 52 ounces (1560 ml) (with more than 42 g of sugar) without even thinking twice and without feeling even slightly full. And while most people understand that soda is really bad for you, many do not understand that there are dozens and dozens of beverages lurking in the supermarket aisles that look healthy, sound healthy, and even taste healthy but are nothing more than lightly dressed up sugar water.

So this chapter is about the best things to drink. But first, full disclosure: I consider sugar—not fat—to be the number-one health challenge facing America. I believe that when all is sorted out—and it may not be in our lifetime—we will discover that sugar is what is fueling the obesity crisis. When the true connection between insulin—the hormone that is raised by eating simple sugars and processed carbs—and Alzheimer's disease, cancer, heart disease, diabetes, and obesity is fully understood, we will finally understand that fat has far less to do with our health outcomes than sugar, and never really did. But that's a long, long way off from being accepted knowledge. I mention it so that you know my bias, and you know where I stand. What I've tried to do in this chapter is find the best things to drink that will give you the largest nutritional bang for the buck with the absolute least amount of insulin-raising sugar in the bargain.

Fortunately, many beverages meet that standard. Let's say hello.

RED WINE

Red wine is a great drink for two reasons (and not such a great drink for one or two other reasons). First the good stuff: alcohol and polyphenols.

A substantial amount of epidemiological evidence links moderate consumption of alcohol with reduced risk for heart disease. Moderate drinking seems to be good for the circulatory system and may—in some way not fully understood—offer some protection against diabetes and gallstones. Moderate consumers of alcohol have fewer heart attacks and strokes, are likely to live longer than abstainers, and are generally less likely to have high blood pressure, Alzheimer's disease, and even the common cold. This is true across the board of moderate alcohol consumption regardless of whether it's from wine or spirits.

But red wine has a special added benefit. It contains polyphenols—plant compounds with health benefits—specifically one superstar polyphenol

Alcohol: Men and Women Are Not Alike

Men and women process alcohol very, very differently. Get over it. It's a fact, and you need to understand this difference. Here's why.

While it may be true that moderate drinking is associated with a reduced rate of heart disease, even moderate—I'm talking one drink a day—drinking for women increases the risk of breast cancer by 12 percent or so. That doesn't mean that if you drink you have a 12 percent chance of getting cancer. But it does mean that if 10 women in 100 were going to get it, drinking raises the odds to a little more than 11 women in 100. You don't want to be that extra one, and here's how to make sure you're not: Take folic acid.

The increased risk disappears in women who are not low on folic acid. I think everyone should be taking folic acid anyway, but now you have an extra reason to do so. There's a really great liquid form of folic acid in an eyedropper that I like a lot called Super Liquid Folate, which makes it easy and painless to take it daily, and it comes with some B12, which is a good idea for many reasons. You can find a link to it on the shopping section of my website, www.jonnybowden.com. Or take a good multivitamin that contains at least 400—and preferably 800—mcg of the stuff.

called resveratrol, which is currently under investigation for its presumed antiaging effects. Resveratrol is one of the most potent polyphenols, and it's found in both red wine and the seeds and skins of grapes (as well as a few other foods). Red wine has a high concentration of this powerful antioxidant because the skins and seeds ferment in the grapes' juices during the red wine-making process. This prolonged contact during their fermentation process produces significant levels of resveratrol in the finished red wine.

Resveratrol has an impressive résumé. It's been shown to extend the life span of every life form tested so far, including yeast cells, fruit flies, worms, mice, and probably monkeys. Resveratrol has anticancer activity, exhibiting anticancer properties against a wide range of tumor cells. It may also improve blood flow in the brain by 30 percent, thus reducing the risk of stroke.

But red wine—and all alcohol—has a dark side. According to the National Institute on Alcohol Abuse and Alcoholism (as of 2000):

- 14 million Americans meet standard criteria for alcohol abuse or alcoholism.
- Alcohol plays a role in one in four cases of violent crime.
- More than 16,000 people die each year in automobile accidents in which alcohol was involved.
- Alcohol abuse costs more than 180 billion dollars a year.

So don't start drinking to get the benefits of alcohol and red wine. But if you already are drinking, make it moderate. That's defined as 1 or 2 drinks a day for men and no more than 1 a day for women. In the United States, 1 drink is usually considered to be 12 ounces (355 ml) of beer, 5 ounces (150 ml) of wine, or 1½ ounces (45 ml) of spirits (hard liquor such as gin or whiskey). Each delivers about 12 to 14 g of alcohol.

In the introduction, I discussed the concept of the polymeal, a hypothetical perfect meal designed by researchers that, if eaten daily, would substantially reduce the risk for heart disease as much as or more than many medications. Wine was a part of it. In fact, the authors calculated that based on the available research, 150 ml of wine a day would likely result in a 23 to 41 percent reduction in risk for coronary heart disease.

LIQUID FRUITS

Because most supermarket fruit juices are nothing more than sugar water, I'm not a fan of them. Look closely and you will see ingredients such as high-fructose corn syrup among the first ingredients, which is a particularly dangerous kind of sugar that raises triglycerides and ultimately insulin. Look further and you'll find that many fruit juices are actually fruit "cocktails," and somewhere in the small print will proclaim that they are made with 10 percent of "real fruit juice." Ten percent? You've got to be kidding. None of this stuff is any good, and it certainly doesn't deserve a place at the table of any of the "Healthiest Meals on Earth."

But it is possible to get a reasonably low-sugar, antioxidant-rich juice, and some of these can really be extraordinary for your health. Here are some of my favorite "liquid fruits."

Pomegranate juice: Long-term consumption of pomegranate juice may help slow aging and protect against heart disease and cancer. It contains one of the highest antioxidant capacities of any juice, and it compares favorably to red wine and green tea. At least five studies have demonstrated a beneficial effect of pomegranate juice on cardiovascular health.

Noni juice: Noni juice is expensive, but it appears to have a really rich assortment of phytochemicals that may turn out to have anticancer properties. The science on the Morinda citrifolia fruit (from which noni juice is made) is still evolving, but it looks pretty promising. I add a couple of ounces to my juice and drinks almost daily.

Cranberry juice: It's hard to find the unsweetened stuff—most is cranberry "cocktail" and I've already told you what I think of that—but it's worth looking for. Yes, it's bitter, and yes it's pricey, but if you dilute it with water it lasts a long time. Cranberries are a rich source of antioxidants, plus there are bioactive compounds in whole cranberries that are toxic to a variety of cancer tumor cells. Cranberry juice also helps prevent urinary tract infections. And although I'm not a fan because of the sugar, even the ordinary cranberry juice cocktail has been shown to have a high content of phenols, plant chemicals with multiple health benefits.

Grape juice: Newly published research shows that Concord purple grape juice scores higher in a group of natural plant antioxidants called

Meal Prep Tips

- In general, don't peel, seed, or stem your fruits and vegetables before juicing. Leaving any delicate skins intact will increase the nutrient content of your drink. (You will, however, need to remove pits and peel heavier fruit skins such as banana or citrus fruits.)

- Drink fresh juices shortly after making for maximum nutrient impact.

- Fresh juices, especially green ones, can be powerfully cleansing, so start slowly with small amounts.

- Don't gulp your juice: Sip it slowly, mixing each mouthful with saliva to support its digestion.

proanthocyanidins than any of the other juices or beverages tested on a per serving basis. Proanthocyanidins are part of a larger family of plant compounds known as flavonoids that have been shown to have multiple health benefits. The flavonoids in grape juice have also been shown to prevent the oxidation of so-called bad cholesterol (LDLs, or low-density lipoproteins) that leads to formation of plaque in artery wall.

Here are two important disclaimers: First, avoid "grape drinks" like the plague and look for the real thing: pure juice from real grapes. And second, even though they're rich in healthy plant compounds, both grapes and grape juice have a lot of sugar. If you need to watch your sugar carefully, grape juice may not be a good drink for you.

Black cherry juice: Cherries are loaded with anti-inflammatory, antiaging, anticancer compounds, including a superstar member of the flavonoid family called quercetin. They also contain ellagic acid, which is a naturally occurring plant chemical known to be anticarcinogenic. Cherry juice contains compounds called anthocyanins, which are the pigments that give the fruit its bright red color and are also believed to be the key to cherries' well-known anti-inflammatory actions. For what it's worth, the old-school, contrarian guru of bodybuilding from the '60s and '70s, Vince Gironda, recommended black cherry juice on a daily basis to his bodybuilders. Again, get the unsweetened kind!

GREEN DRINKS

Whenever I've written a story for a popular magazine or website and mentioned green drinks, it's always come back with a note from the editor asking, "What is this?" Understandable. Green drinks are a newly emerging category of beverage that has such a wide definition no one can really agree on exactly what they are. They're kind of in the category of "I know it when I see it." But here are the basics.

Green drinks are usually made from grasses (such as wheatgrass), young barley greens, or blue green algae, and/or they contain a mix of extracts from green plants such as spinach, kale, broccoli, and wheatgrass. They're popping up everywhere. I see ready-made green drinks in small plastic containers in bigger health food stores (with names like "Green Power" and

"Green Essence"). Sometimes they'll add some protein powder for a kind of hybrid drink. And the category of green drinks probably should include juices you make at home in the blender or food processor that have a decidedly green "flavor" or color, even if they include some fruit for flavor.

You can buy "ready-mix" preparations, powders you can mix up with water, such as PaleoGreens. (They're available under "drinks and shakes" on my website, www.jonnybowden.com.) One excellent product available both on my website and in stores is Barlean's Greens.

Jeannette recommends simple green drinks such as wheatgrass (powdered, fresh, or frozen), young barley greens (powdered), and blue green algae (powdered or frozen, especially E3 Live frozen, available at www.e3live.com) "If you can tolerate it," she says, "I recommend drinking these 'straight' and away from other foods, for example in the early morning or as a midafternoon pick-me-up. They're easier to digest when drunk alone and the alkalizing effect is 'undiluted,' very calming and balancing." They are also very cleansing, so if you aren't used to drinking your greens, start with small amounts: a teaspoon at a time with at least eight ounces of water.

SMOOTHIES: THE LIQUID POLYMEAL

There are endless variations on how to make a smoothie, but the purpose of this section is to give you a template from which you can experiment with your own liquid polymeal. Like the polymeal, your smoothie should have as many of the following ingredients as possible: protein, fat, fiber, antioxidants, anti-inflammatories, vitamins, and minerals. By using the five basic ingredients listed on page 339, you'll have the basis for an enormous number of superb-tasting drinks that will provide you with endless benefits and a rich variety of tastes and textures.

Also on page 339, we've listed some of our favorite add-ins. You can really be creative with this; the combinations are endless and also delightful. I remember the first time I discovered that a couple of spoonfuls of oats and a spoonful of almond or peanut butter went beautifully in a basic protein shake of protein powder and berries. There really are no rules; have fun with this.

Smoothie Season?

Some people stop making smoothies in the colder months because they think they need to be frozen or really, really cold. We naturally shy away from colder dishes and drinks in the winter season, especially in the morning. But you can happily make them all year round: Some smoothies are fantastic at room temperature. The Hunger Buster and Nut Power, for example, make great winter smoothies because they taste their best at room temperature.

Sultry Summer Sangria
The pitcher of heart health

Ingredients

1 bottle good red wine, such as Merlot, Cabernet Sauvignon, or a Spanish Rioja

1 lemon, cut into quarters, quarters halved into wedges

1 lime, cut into quarters, quarters halved into wedges

1 orange, cut into quarters, quarters halved into wedges

1 cup (145 g) strawberries, stemmed and sliced

2 ripe kiwifruit, peeled and sliced

½ cup (80 g) fresh pineapple chunks

1 tablespoon (15 ml) fresh pineapple juice

½ cup (120 ml) orange juice

2 tablespoons (28 ml) ginger juice

2 tablespoons (40 g) agave nectar, or more if you like it sweeter

¼ to ½ cup (60 to 120 ml) ginger brandy

4 cups (about 1 L) plain seltzer

Pour the wine into a large pitcher. Gently squeeze the wedges of lemon, lime, and orange into the wine, removing the seeds when possible. (Do not squeeze all the juices out.) Place the fruit wedges into the wine. Add the strawberries, kiwi, and pineapple chunks. Gently stir the pineapple juice, orange juice, and ginger juice into the wine. Add the agave nectar and brandy and stir. Gently pour the seltzer in and stir once or twice lightly to mix. Refrigerate overnight. Serve anytime the next day right from the pitcher or in a punch bowl.

Yield: About 8 to 9 servings

Notes from the Kitchen

- You will need to let this chill and marinate in the refrigerator overnight before serving.

- This sangria recipe is not nearly as sweet as what you may be used to. There is no need to load sangria down with ginger ale and buckets of sugar to get a tasty, satisfying cocktail. In fact, you can ditch the soda and sugar entirely. The fruit, wine, and simple spices make this drink warm and delicious on its own, with a clean pleasant bite. It's a perfect drink for a summer evening party, and don't forget to enjoy the marinated fruit!

- Sangria is a drink that you can have a lot of fun making because it lends itself well to experimentation. The main components are the wine, fruit, and seltzer. Try different combinations of fruits and play with the additions of other spices (how about whole cloves or cinnamon sticks?) and liquors (peach brandy? cinnamon schnapps?). Avoid wines that are too oaky.

- You really need to use organic citrus fruit in this recipe because the peels (where the bulk of the pesticides dwell) will be marinating in the wine all night long. And even though the fruit is organic, be sure to scrub it with a brush before using to get it really clean.

- To make the ginger juice, peel and grate fresh ginger to make 3 to 4 tablespoons (24 to 32 g) of ginger gratings. Squeeze the gratings to extract the juice.

- Many of these smoothie recipes call for unsweetened, unflavored almond milk and whey protein powder. We suggest using these as a base because we think they are the best nutritional choices with virtually no sugars, clean digestible protein, and a small amount of healthy fats. But if you prefer, you can use any of the other suggested milks, such as rice or cow, or proteins, such as rice or hemp, in their stead.

Liver Support
Drink up for detox

½ cucumber

1 carrot

½ cup (30 g) packed parsley

3 stalks celery

¼ lime

Wash the cucumber, carrot, parsley, and celery very well and shake to dry.

Slice the cucumber half in half lengthwise so it will fit easily into the juicer's feeder.

Juice the cucumber and carrot. Juice the parsley and finish with the celery. Squeeze the lime into the juice, stir gently, and enjoy.

Yield: 1 serving

Jonny's Recipe for Supermarket SuperJuice
An anti-aging, anti-cancer, anti-inflammatory superstar

2 ounces (60 ml) unsweetened noni juice

2 ounces (60 ml) unsweetened black cherry juice

2 ounces (60 ml) unsweetened cranberry juice

4 to 6 ounces (120 to 175 ml) unsweetened pomegranate juice

10 to 12 ounces (285 to 355 ml) water

Xylitol, optional

In a tall glass, pour the noni juice, black cherry juice, cranberry juice, pomegranate juice, and water to taste. Sweeten with xylitol to taste if desired. Sip throughout the day

Notes from the Kitchen

- When adding nuts or seeds such as pumpkin seeds (which is a great idea!), it helps to soak the raw nuts or seeds in water overnight. It's not absolutely necessary, but it does soften them, starts the sprouting process (converting fat into protein), and definitely makes them more digestible.

- I have found the best oil to use is MCT oil. (MCT, you may recall, stands for medium-chain triglycerides, which are a type of fat in the saturated fat family that are actually very beneficial to the body and have a number of health benefits.) It's virtually tasteless, so it gives the smoothie a frothy texture but without the overbearing, and often generally yucky, taste of fish or flaxseed oils. Plus, you don't have to worry about the whole deal with having men avoid flax oil.

Liquid Polymeal Formula
A starting point for personalized smoothies

1 cup (235 ml) milk, such as cow, almond, or rice

1 scoop protein powder (whey, egg protein, hemp, rice); ⅓ cup (75 g) silken tofu; or ⅓ cup (80 ml) pasteurized egg whites (see "A Good Egg" on page 277 for a discussion about raw eggs)

1 cup (140-170 g) fruit or vegetable, such as fresh or frozen berries, melon, kiwifruit, cherries, papaya, guava, mango, or peaches, or 1 to 2 tablespoons (13 g) cranberries (with a sweetener), or ⅓ cup (75 g) cooked pumpkin or skinned baked sweet potato

1 to 2 tablespoons (15–30 ml) great fats, such as avocado, flaxseed oil, coconut milk, coconut oil, almonds, pecans, cashews, sunflower seeds, pumpkin seeds, or nut butters, or 1 teaspoon fish oil

1 to 2 tablespoons (7–14 g) extra fiber, such as ground flaxseed or flax meal, raw whole oats, wheat germ or bran, or a fiber supplement such as FiberSmart

Optional extras, to taste, such as dried coconut, dried goji berries, prunes, maca powder, fresh bee pollen, raw cacao, cinnamon, cardamom, pumpkin pie spice, nutmeg, nutritional yeast, powdered ginger, ginger juice, ⅓ banana, 1 teaspoon to 1 tablespoon (20 g) agave nectar or raw honey, sprinkling xylitol, or 1 packet or 2 drops stevia

Place all of the ingredients in a blender and process until smooth.

Yield: 1 generous or 2 small servings

Hunger Buster

Satisfy your appetite for omegas-3s

1 cup (235 ml) almond milk

1 scoop whey protein powder

½ cup (115 g) baked, chilled, and peeled yam

½ juicy orange, peeled and seeded

1 tablespoon (15 ml) Barlean's Omega Twin oil or any flaxseed oil

1 tablespoon (15 g) raw rolled oats (not quick cooking)

½ teaspoon ground cinnamon

Place the milk, protein powder, yam, orange, oil, oats, and cinnamon in a blender. Blend everything together well and serve.

Yield: 1 large or 2 small smoothies

Notes from the Kitchen

- The yam tastes better when it's been cooked and then chilled in the fridge versus hot out of the oven!

Sweet Morning Eye Opener

A digestive delight

2 carrots

1 red apple, such as Red Delicious, Fuji, or Pink Lady

1-inch-square (3-cm-square) peeled chunk fresh ginger, or more if you like it hot

Scrub the carrots and apple. Cut the apple into quarters so it fits easily into the juicer's feeder. Place the carrot, apple, and ginger into the juicer, juice everything, stir it gently, and enjoy.

The Best Little Beverage in the World

A healthiest meals book would not be complete without at least a mention of a beverage that can accompany any meal on the planet (and frequently does): tea.

Though green tea gets the lion's share of the attention, truth be told all four kinds of nonherbal tea—green, black, white, and oolong (red)—come from the same plant, camellia sinensis. They differ only by the degree of processing and fermentation, but all of them offer major health benefits.

All teas contain polyphenols, which are powerful antioxidants, many of which have anticancer activities. Polyphenols help protect the cells (and your DNA) from damage known as oxidative stress. And although the teas differ somewhat in terms of what plant chemicals they contain, there's not a bad one in the lot.

And here's a tip for you. A new kid on the tea block, yerba matte, which comes from a whole different plant, is being researched for its powerful antioxidant properties. In one study, it was found to have more antioxidant power than any of the other four teas. It makes a great addition to your tea collection.

According to the excellent book *The Story of Tea: A Cultural History and Drinking Guide* by Mary Lou Heiss and Bob Heiss, the perfect cup of tea requires pretty exact steeping times and temperatures.

- Black tea: 3 to 5 minutes at 190°F (88°C) to 200°F (93°C)
- Oolong tea: 90 seconds to 2 minutes at 180°F (82°C) to 200°F (93°C)
- White tea: 90 seconds to 2 minutes at 160°F (71°C) to 170°F (77°C)
- Standard green tea: 2 to 3 minutes at 170°F (77°C) to 180°F (82°C)
- Japanese green tea: 2 to 3 minutes at 160°F (71°C) to 170°F (77°C)
- Spring or new green tea: 90 seconds to 2 minutes at 160°F (71°C) to 170°F (77°C)
- Pu-erh tea: 2 to 5 minutes at 200°F (93°C) to 212°F (100°C)

Frozen Tropical Treat
Fabulous fat and fiber

Ingredients

1 cup (235 ml) almond milk, well chilled

1 scoop whey protein powder

½ ripe peach, peeled, or ½ cup (85 g) frozen peach slices

⅓ frozen banana, peeled (see page 131)

¼ cup (40 g) fresh or frozen pineapple chunks

1 frozen coconut milk "ice cube" (about a generous tablespoon see page 131)

1 tablespoon (7 g) FiberSmart

1 tablespoon (15 ml) pure cranberry juice (not concentrated!)

1 tablespoon (5 g) dried unsweetened coconut

Place the milk, protein powder, peach, banana, pineapple, coconut milk "ice cube," FiberSmart, cranberry juice, and coconut in a blender. Blend everything together well and serve.

Yield: 1 large or 2 small smoothies

The Whole Fruit and Nothing but the Fruit

If you are a real smoothie fan, Jeannette and I strongly recommend investing in a powerful, well-made blender. We both own and love our Vita-Mix. It has an engine like a lawn mower and can handle anything thrown into it.

Jeannette writes, "I know these machines are pricey, but over the years I've found that my higher-quality components such as the Vita-Mix blender or my KitchenAid mixer rarely, if ever, need to be repaired or replaced. They require an initial investment, but if you, like me, use your kitchen hard—and I truly hope you do—they are well worth the cost."

I agree. At my house, we periodically go for a day or three living on a rich, liquefied mix of broccoli, cucumber, apples, carrots, beets, celery, and peeled avocado (including the pit, which is a rich source of nutrients), all of which are easily liquefied by these superjuicers. You can even throw in a whole egg, shell and all. This way you lose none of the fiber.

Melon Snap

A sweet load of potassium

1 cup (235 ml) almond milk

1 scoop whey protein powder

½ cup (80 g) fresh or frozen melon, such as honeydew
   or cantaloupe

½ cup (80 g) fresh or frozen mango

1 tablespoon (7 g) ground flaxseed

1 tablespoon (15 ml) ginger juice

Place the milk, protein powder, melon, mango, flaxseed, and ginger juice in a blender. Blend everything together well and serve.

Yield: 1 large or 2 small smoothies

Note from the Kitchen

- To make 1 tablespoon (15 ml) fresh ginger juice, peel and grate fresh ginger to get 1 to 2 tablespoons (8 to 16 g) gratings. Squeeze the gratings to extract the juice.

Nut Power

Power up with plenty of fiber and protein

1 cup (235 ml) almond milk

1 scoop whey protein powder

1 small ripe banana, peeled

2 tablespoons (32 g) raw almond butter

1 tablespoon (7 g) FiberSmart

1 teaspoon dried maca powder

Place the milk, protein powder, banana, almond butter, FiberSmart, and maca powder in a blender. Blend everything together well and serve.

Yield: 1 large or 2 small smoothies

Functional Foods and Beverages: Do You Really Need Gingko Tea?

Lately, there's been a virtual explosion of drinks in what could loosely be called the "energy drink" category. Technically, the industry calls these "functional foods," a very (very) loose category that encompasses any food or beverage that is supposed to have a health benefit beyond just what you would expect from eating (or drinking) it. For example, you can buy orange juice fortified with calcium for strong bones, yogurt with acidophilus for better digestion, and pasta with added omega-3s for heart and brain health.

So far, so good. But recently, the category has expanded all over the place, with all sorts of "enriched" teas and drinks that trade on the reputation of the added ingredient and hope you don't notice that there's not much of it in there. For example there are gingko teas, vitamin waters, and iced teas with added carnitine or coenzyme Q10.

Here's the bottom line: Save your money.

The ingredients—gingko, carnitine, CoQ10, and the like—are just fine. There's good research on all of them, showing that they do great things. (See my book *The Most Effective Natural Cures on Earth*.) The problem is that these manufacturers put infinitesimal amounts of these ingredients into an average beverage and hope you won't know (or notice) that the dose is nowhere near the amount needed to produce any real benefit. In fact, if I were being cynical, I'd say that the only reason they add these things in is so they can say their products contain the respected ingredient and so they can charge you more money for it.

You're better off drinking a "nonenhanced" beverage and using the money you save to buy the supplements you want in the dosages that matter.

Antioxidants on the Run
Free-radical roundup

Ingredients

1½ cups (220 g) fresh or frozen
strawberries, or other berries, or a
combo

⅓ cup (80 ml) lightly pasteurized raw
egg whites

1 tablespoon (15 ml) flaxseed oil

1 packet or a few drops stevia, to taste

Place the berries, egg whites, oil, and stevia in a blender. Blend everything together until it's whipped into a light frothy drink and serve.

Yield: 1 large or 2 small smoothies

Notes from the Kitchen

- This smoothie doesn't follow the formula. It's simpler for times when you're in a real hurry. It's great as a workout snack.

- The reason we aren't using the yolks here is not nutritional, but rather for looks and taste. The egg whites give the smoothie its light whipped consistency. The smoothie wouldn't work as well if we included the yolk. Also, whole raw eggs are harder to pasteurize. See page 277 for more information about eating raw eggs.

Chapter 14 **Pantry List**

FOOD GROUP	FOOD	RECIPE
Dairy	Egg whites	Antioxidants on the Run
	Milk (cow, almond or rice)	Liquid Polymeal Formula
Grains	Rolled oats (raw)	Hunger Buster
Herbs/Spices/ Condiments	Cinnamon (ground)	Hunger Buster
	Ginger (fresh)	Sweet Morning Eye Opener
	Ginger juice	Melon Snap, Sultry Summer Sangria
	Parsley (fresh)	Liver Support: The Alkalizer
Miscellaneous	Agave nectar	Sultry Summer Sangria
	Dried maca powder	Nut Power
	Oil/Fats (avocado, flaxseed oil, coconut milk, coconut oil, almonds, pecans, cashews, sunflower seeds, pumpkin seeds, nut butters, or fish oil)	Liquid Polymeal Formula
	FiberSmart	Frozen Tropical Treat, nut Power
	Ginger brandy	Sultry Summer Sangria
	Extra fiber (ground flaxseed or flax meal, raw whole oats, wheat germ or bran)	Liquid Polymeal Formula
	Protein powder (or tofu or egg whites)	Liquid Polymeal Formula
	Whey, protein powder	Frozen Tropical Treat, Hunger Buster, Melon Snap, Nut Power
	Red wine	Sultry Summer Sangria
	Seltzer	Sultry Summer Sangria
	Stevia	Antioxidants on the Run
	Xylitol	Jonny's Recipe for Supermarket SuperJuice
Nuts/Seeds	Almond butter	Nut Power
	Almond milk	Frozen Tropical Treat, Hunger Buster, Melon Snap, Nut Power
	Coconut (dried)	Frozen Tropical Treat
	Coconut milk	Frozen Tropical Treat
	Flaxseed	Melon Snap
	Flaxseed oil	Antioxidants on the Run, Hunger Buster

FOOD GROUP	FOOD	RECIPE
Produce	Apple (red)	Sweet Morning Eye Opener
	Banana	Frozen Tropical Treat, Nut Power
	Black cherry juice	Jonny's Recipe for Supermarket SuperJuice
	Carrot	Liver Support: The Alkalizer, Sweet Morning Eye Opener
	Celery	Liver Support: The Alkalizer
	Cranberry juice	Frozen Tropical Treat, Jonny's Recipe for Supermarket SuperJuice
	Cucumber	Liver Support: The Alkalizer
	Fruit or vegetable (berries, melon, kiwifruit, cherries, papaya, guava, mango, peaches, cranberries, pumpkin, or sweet potato)	Liquid Polymeal Formula
	Kiwifruit	Sultry Summer Sangria
	Lemon	Sultry Summer Sangria
	Lime	Liver Support: The Alkalizer, Sultry Summer Sangria
	Mango (fresh or frozen)	Melon Snap
	Melon (fresh or frozen)	Melon Snap
	Noni (juice)	Jonny's Recipe for Supermarket SuperJuice
	Orange	Hunger Buster, Sultry Summer Sangria
	Orange juice	Sultry Summer Sangria
	Peach (fresh or frozen)	Frozen Tropical Treat
	Pineapple	Frozen Tropical Treat, Sultry Summer Sangria
	Pineapple juice	Sultry Summer Sangria
	Pomegranate juice	Jonny's Recipe for Supermarket SuperJuice
	Strawberries	Antioxidants on the Run, Sultry Summer Sangria
	Yam	Hunger Buster

Food Chart of the Healthiest Ingredients on Earth

On the following chart you can see at a glance some of the documented health benefits of more than sixty foods.

Though not every single ingredient in *The Healthiest Meals on Earth* is listed, most of them are. We left out the "big protein" foods like turkey, chicken, grass-fed meat, and wild salmon—not because they don't matter. They most certainly do. But their primary purpose is to provide protein, a few minerals and vitamins (especially the Bs), plus, of course, in the case of the wild fish, omega-3 fats. It's the plant foods in the chart, however, that are the heavyweights when it comes to antioxidants, fiber, anti-inflammatories, and phytochemicals, and these are the ones we wanted to concentrate on for the purposes of this chart.

Not every single ingredient in every meal in the book wound up in the chart—it's more a reference guide to important health properties of major plant foods than it is a definitive guide to all ingredients in *The Healthiest Meals on Earth*. Similarly, some foods that made the chart aren't actually in any recipes, but they might make terrific substitutions or additions. The point wasn't necessarily to provide an encyclopedia of foods and their uses (for that—if you will excuse the shameless plug—please read *The 150 Healthiest Foods on Earth*)!

The point was to give you a simple, easy-to-use chart in which you could see at a glance all the wonderful things these plant foods can do for you (and your family).

Two acknowledgments are due: My friend, Kathy Barnett, R.N., a registered nurse and health educator with a passion for nutrition and health, originally gave me the idea for this chart and provided a very valuable template. My brilliant assistants, Suzanne Copp, M.S., and Susan Mudd, M.S., C.N.S., pored over a ton of published nutrition research to "vet" (and substantiate) every single entry and validate their "claims to fame." Thanks, guys. I hope you refer to this chart often and that it inspires you to make all the foods on it a part of your own personal "polymeal" plan.

	Cancer Protection	Heart Healthy	Lowers Blood Pressure	Lowers Cholesterol	Promotes Blood Sugar Balance	Protects Bones	Fortifies Vision	Supports Healthy Digestion
Almonds	●	●		●	●			
Apples	●	●		●		●		
Artichokes		●		●	●			●
Asparagus	●	●						
Avocados			●	●				
Bananas						●		●
Beans	●	●		●	●			●
Beets	●	●		●				
Blueberries	●	●			●		●	●
Brazil nuts	●	●						
Broccoli	●	●	●			●	●	
Brussels sprouts	●	●						●
Cabbage	●	●						●
Cantaloupe	●	●	●				●	
Carrots	●	●					●	●
Cashews	●	●		●		●		
Cauliflower	●	●						
Celery	●	●	●					●
Cherries	●	●						
Chestnuts		●		●				
Chili peppers	●			●				●
Coconut		●						
Cranberries	●	●						●
Dandelion			●		●	●		
Eggs	●		●				●	
Figs		●	●					
Fish	●	●	●	●				
Flax	●	●			●			●
Garlic	●	●	●	●				
Grapefruit	●	●		●				
Grapes	●	●					●	
Green tea	●	●						
Guava	●	●	●					

	Cancer Protection	Heart Healthy	Lowers Blood Pressure	Lowers Cholesterol	Promotes Blood Sugar Balance	Protects Bones	Fortifies Vision	Supports Healthy Digestion
Kale	●	●					●	
Kiwifruit	●	●						
Lemons	●	●						
Limes	●	●						
Mangoes	●	●						
Mushrooms	●	●						
Oats	●	●		●	●			●
Olive oil	●	●		●	●			
Onions	●	●		●	●			●
Oranges	●	●	●	●				●
Papaya	●	●		●			●	●
Peaches	●	●					●	●
Peanuts		●	●	●	●			
Pecans		●		●		●		
Pineapple	●			●		●	●	●
Pomegranate	●	●		●				
Prunes	●	●		●	●			●
Pumpkin	●	●			●		●	●
Raspberries	●						●	
Rice (brown)	●						●	●
Spinach	●		●	●	●	●	●	
Strawberries	●	●					●	
Sunflower seeds	●		●	●	●	●		
Sweet potatoes	●	●						
Swiss chard	●	●				●	●	
Tomatoes	●	●	●			●		●
Walnuts	●	●	●	●	●			●
Water	●	●	●					●
Watercress	●	●				●		
Watermelon	●	●	●	●			●	
Wheat bran	●	●		●				●
Wheat germ	●	●		●				●
Whey protein	●	●		●	●			
Yogurt	●			●		●		●

The Right Oil for the Job

Confused about which oil to reach for in the kitchen? The chart on pages 356 and 357 will give you some ideas. High-quality oils can provide a rich source of different types of healthy fat, a crucial component of the polymeal. But it's important to know a bit about each of them so that you can choose the right oil for your dishes.

Many oils are quite fragile, meaning that heat can break them down and change their structure. Some oils, the most delicate, cannot be subjected to heat at all. These oils, such as flax and fish, need to be kept in the refrigerator and enjoyed cold. Other oils, such as almond and avocado, remain quite stable even at very high temperatures. They are the best ones to use for any type of high-heat cooking, such as searing or broiling.

The temperature at which oil begins to break down is called its smoke point, so you want to keep each oil below its smoke point at all times. If you do overheat oil and it begins to smoke in the pan, simply empty and wash the pan and start again with a fresh batch at a lower temperature. There is some disagreement as to the precise smoke points for different oils, so in this chart we offer you smoke points erring on the lower side, rather than the higher side, for safety.

An Overhyped Oil

If you're looking for an oil and don't see it on the chart, then it just didn't make the cut as a healthy oil, and you may be surprised at some that didn't.

Canola oil, for instance, has been widely advocated as a healthy choice, but contrary to popular belief, canola oil is not a preferred choice. It's an overhyped and unhealthy oil that has undeservingly reaped the benefits of great marketing by the oil industry. As the esteemed lipid biochemist Mary Enig, Ph.D., points out, "Like all modern vegetable oils, canola oil goes through the process of caustic refining, bleaching, and degumming—all of which involve high temperatures of questionable safety."

The wonderful omega-3s in canola oil easily become rancid when subjected to the high temperature needed to extract the canola oil. Therefore, they have to be deodorized. This deodorizing process turns a large number of the omega-3s into trans fats. And canola oil used in foods is even worse, as it hydrogenates beautifully, making it ideal for shelf life but not for your life, as the hydrogenation just increases the trans fat content.

So if you're looking for canola, safflower, grapeseed, or other oils on this list and don't see them, there was a reason for it. For some of you, it may be time for an oil change.

No matter what oil you reach for, here are some basic guidelines to remember:

- Use cold storage for oils. Oils should be stored in opaque or dark containers and away from heat. Keeping them in the fridge is a good option and will guarantee protection against any free radical formation.

- Take a multivitamin with your oils. Because oils consist of delicate carbon chains, they can go rancid pretty easily. Another name for rancidity is free radicals, which destroy cells. A good antioxidant will help to stem the progression of free radicals, so remember to take a multivitamin if you are not eating an antioxidant-rich meal that contains, for example, dark greens or colorful fruits and berries.

- Look for cold-pressed on the label. Cold-pressed means that the oil was not subjected to commercial heating and processing, which offers greater protection against free radical formation.

The Right Oil for the Job

OIL	HEAT	PRIMARY TYPE OF OIL	SMOKE POINT
Almond*	High	Monounsaturated	430°F (221°C)
Avocado*	High	Monounsaturated	510°F (266°C)
Clarified butter (ghee)*	Medium-high	Saturated	350°F (180°C)
Coconut *	Medium-high	90 percent saturated	350°F (180°C)
Fish *	No	Polyunsaturated	n/a
Flaxseed*	Low/no	Polyunsaturated	225°F (107°C)
Hempseed	Medium	Polyunsaturated	330°F (165°C)
Macadamia nut *	Medium-high	Monounsaturated	390°F (195°C)
Olive*	Medium	Monounsaturated	Unrefined extra virgin: 320°F (160°C)
Peanut	Medium	Monounsaturated, some polyunsaturated and saturated	Refined, 450°F (230°C); Unrefined, 320°F (160°C)
Sesame	Medium	Monounsaturated and polyunsaturated	Refined, 410°F (210°C); Unrefined, 350°F (180°C)
Walnut	Medium	Polyunsaturated	320°F (160°C)

* These oils can be found in recipes throughout this book.

FLAVOR	IDEAL FOR	HEALTH BENEFITS
Nutty	Sautéing, stir-frying, searing, baking	High in omega-3 essential fatty acids
Mild, neutral	Making popcorn	High in vitamins A, B1, B2, D, and E
Slight nutty flavor	Any type of cooking	Enhances digestion
Mild, distinct odor	Baking	Antiviral, antibacterial properties
Fishy	Protein shakes	Reduces cholesterol and inflammation
Nutty	Drizzle on salads or vegetables	Highest plant source of omega-3s
Mild, nutty	Salads, protein shakes, and vegetable juices	Rich in essential fatty acids
Mellow, nutty flavor	Salads	High in antioxidants and vitamin D
Neutral	Salads, cooking (do not use extra virgin for cooking: heat will create free radicals)	High in antioxidants
Peanut	Stir-fying, sautéing	Resistant to rancidity
Sesame	Stir-fying, asian salads	High in vitamin E, detoxifying properties
Walnut	Drizzle on salads and vegetables	High in omega-3 fatty acids

Sources for Specialty Ingredients

Great resource for ordering organic/free-range/grass-fed animal and plant foods, including buffalo, turkey, and dairy. They even have a terrific raw selection.
www.diamondorganics.com

Good resource for ordering venison and other wild game meats:
http://brokenarrowranch.com

Good resource for ordering calf's liver:
www.azulunabrands.com

Good resource for raw foods, including goji berries, cacao powder, and agave nectar:
www.rawfoods.com

For a nice selection of artisan vinegars:
www.chefshop.com/items.asp?Cc=VINEGAR&tp=

For the fabulous Minus 8 vinegar source:
http://minus8vinegar.com

For Barlean's terrific line of flax products, coconut oil, and other omega products:
www.barleans.com

For Sprinkle Fiber product:
www.fiberdiet35.com/SprinkleFiber.html

For E3 Live frozen blue green algae:
www.e3live.com

For raw organic honey:
www.reallyrawhoney.com

For wild salmon and other really pure fish:
www.vitalchoice.com

For organic, grass-fed beef and meat products from a family farm:
www.uswellnessmeats.com

You can also order grass-fed meats and wild salmon through links on my website under "Shopping" then "Healthy Foods":
www.jonnybowden.com

Acknowledgments

We wish to thank the many folks who contributed to this book in countless different ways. We are deeply grateful for all your support and multiple talents! You helped this project come to life.

To Cara Connors, editor extraordinaire: You made it easy and fun—a rare experience on a complex book. Thank you for your tireless work, golden feedback, and endless positive attitude. To Jennifer Bright Reich: Thank you for clear and thoughtful editorial support—you helped us better write what we truly wanted to say! And to Catrine Kelty, food stylist; Rosalind Wanke, creative director; Daria Perreault, art director; and Glenn Scott, photographer, thank you for the gorgeous images. And, of course, many thanks to our agent, the indefatigable Coleen O'Shea, clearly the best agent on earth, and a food lover to boot. What a combo.

To the Spectacular Sues—Suzanne Copp, M.S., and Susan Mudd, M.S., C.N.S.—you epitomize that wonderful combination of knowledge and wit. Thanks for all your good-natured hard work, especially in the hairy home stretch!

To the recipe contributors Dana Carpender, Christine MacFarlane, traditional naturopath Linda Page, Ph.D., Sophia Pendergast, Andy Rubman, Regina Wilshire, Tracee Yablon-Brenner, and especially Lora Ruffner: Thank you for your great ideas and delicious inspirations!

To the Tasters Team: the Kerr crew, the Paris tribe, Jeannette's mom, Judie Porter, grandmom, Jeannette Porter, whose decades of home cooking continue to inspire and nourish her, and especially to her great friend Ray Cournoyer, who has an excellent palate! Thank you all for your honest and friendly feedback.

Jonny: To my darling Anja and our two dogs, Woodstock and Emily, for never once complaining about my cooking.

Jeannette: To my husband Jay and our children, Jesse and Julian, the loves of my life, thank you for your constant humor and patience at the dinner table.

Index

Note: Locators in italics indicate photographs.

A

ACE inhibitors, 305
acetylcholine, 158. *See also* choline
acid-alkaline balance, 308–309
acids, 308–309
acne, 49
ADHD (Attention Deficit Hyperactivity Disorder), 71
advanced glycation end-products (AGES), 250
Agatston, Arthur, 177
agave nectar, 43, 64, 65, 113, 190, 191, 211, 215, 313, 322, 348
AGES. *See* advanced glycation end-products (AGES)
aging, 119, 272, 331
ALA. *See* alpha-linolenic acid
albacore tuna, 121
alcohol, 64, 190, 329, 330. *See also* beer; beverages; wine
alcoholism, 329–330
alkalines, 308–309
Alkalizer, the, *326*, 327, 338, *338*
All Bran, 111
allergies, 88, 95
allicin, 105
allspice, 183, 249, 322
allyl isothiocyanate, 218
allyl sulfides, 249
almond butter, 113, *152*, 153, 158, 168–169, *169*, 171, *326*, 327, 344, *344*, 348
almond extract, 171
almond milk, 113, *114*, 115, 119, 130–131, *131*, 133, 190, 191, *326*, 327, 340, *340*, 342–343, *343*, *344*, 344, 348
almond oil, 129, 133, 205, 211, 267, 274, 356–357
almonds, 9, 11, 17, 65, 190, 211, 267, 309, 348, 352. *See also* almond butter; almond milk; almond oil
Steamed Green Veggies and Nuts, *244*, 245, 258–259, *259*
Sweet Potato Pie with Almond Oat Crust, *212*, 213, 214–215, 218, 236–238, *237*
alpha-linolenic acid (ALA), 69, 71, 303
Alzheimer's disease, 13, 46, 71, 157, 196, 329
amaranth, 309
Amino Acid Score, 155
amino acids, 196, 197, 252, 265, 306
anchovy paste, 297
anthocyanins, 156, 332
antibacterials, 117, 198, 253, 276
antibiotics, 47, 49, 74, 99, 179, 219, 250
antifungals, 198, 253
anti-inflammatories, 10, 14, 17, 71, 88, 94, 156, 178, 195, 198, 248, 275, 303, 332
antimicrobials, 198, 270
antimutagenics, 253
antioxidants, 10, 14, 17, 77, 98, 118, 137–138, 155–156, 176, 195, 196–197, 247, 253, 270, 271, 272, 330, 331, 331–332, 341, 355
Antioxidants on the Run, *326*, 327, 346–347, *347*
antiparasitics, 253, 270
antivirals, 117, 270, 276
aphrodisiacs, 197
apoptosis, 218
apple cider vinegar, 155, 156–157, 171, 323
apples, 42, 110, 177–178, 190, 191, 216, 248, 267, 309, 349, 352
Baked Apples, *172*, 173, 177, 178, 188–189, *189*
cardiovascular health and, 195
Holiday Waldorf Salad, *212*, 213, 215, 216, 218, 232–233, *233*
pesticides on, 248
Sweet Morning Eye Opener, *326*, 327, *340*, 340
types of, 189
apricots, 11, *152*, 153, 158, 168–169, *169*, 171
Armstrong, Lance, 21
artherosclerosis, 117, 275
arthritis, 94, 156
artichokes, 352
artificial ingredients, 99, 159
arugula, 300, 301, 305, 316–317, *317*, 323
ascorbic acid, 88. *See also* vitamin C
asian mustard, 89
asparagus, 42, 211, 267, 309, 352
Asparagus-Endive Salad, *192*, 193, 196, 197, 198, 206–207, *207*
Roasted Brussels Sprouts, Asparagus, and Broccoli with Toasted Hazelnuts, *212*, 213, 215, 217, 218, 230–231, *231*
Steamed Green Veggies and Nuts, *244*, 245, 258–259, *259*
Asparagus-Endive Salad, *192*, 193, 196, 197, 198, 206–207, *207*
aspartame, 159
astaxanthin, 74, 118
asthma, 88, 195
Atkins diet, 13
Attention Deficit Hyperactivity Disorder. *See* ADHD
avocado oil, 65, 356–357
avocados, 12, 13, 42, 43, 136–137, 151, 209, 211, 348, 352
avocado oil, 65, 356–357
Citrus Avocado Salad with Nut Oil, 29, 38–39
fats in, 136–137
Florida vs. California, 137
preparation of, 39
ripening, 39
Ayurvedic medicine, 94

B

B vitamins, 155, 196. *See also* B6; folic acid (vitamin B9); niacin (vitamin B3); pantothenic acid (vitamin B5); riboflavin (vitamin B2); *specific vitamins*; vitamin B12
baby peas, 267. *See also* peas
Baby Spinach Salad with Fresh Raspberries, *44*, 45, 48, 58–59, *59*
bacon. *See* turkey bacon
bacteria, 30, 49, 112, 117, 215, 248, 249, 270, 274, 307. *See also* probiotics
Baked Apples, *172*, 173, 177, 178, 188–189, *189*
baking powder, 65
baking soda, 322
balsamic vinegar, 171
bananas, 42, 88, 113, 125, 133, 209, 211, 277, 349, 352
Nut Power, *326*, 327, 344, *344*
Tropical Frosties, *114*, 115, 119, 130–131, *131*
Barlean's products, 118, 157, 167, 190, 313
barley, 321, 332, 333
barley greens, 332, 333
Barnett, Kathy, 351
basil, 138, 151, 183, 249, 296
Lemon-Herb Salad, *268*, 269, 282–283, *283*
Schlemmertopf-Roasted Pesto Chicken, *268*, 269, 270, 276, 280–281, *281*
basmati rice, 25, 30, 36–37, 43, 296. *See also* rice
bass, *134*, 135, 139, 142–143, *143*, 151
bay leaf, 183, 249, 266, 296
bean curd. *See* tofu
Beano, 31
beans, 27, 28, 28–29, 31, 34–35, 35, 41, 43, 291, 305–306, 309, 352. *See also* lentils; *specific beans*
beef, 266, 309
cuts of, 198
herbs for, 249
Red Beans, Brown Rice, and Lean Beef, *244*, 245, 251–253, 264–265, *265*
spices for, 249
veal, 132
beer, 297, 309
beet greens, *152*, 153, 157, 158, 164–165, *165*, 171
beets, 155, 157, 171, 309, 352. *See also* beet greens
in betaine, 157
cardiovascular health, 157
in folate, 157
liver health and, 157
in potassium, 157
Sweet Beets and Greens, *152*, 153, 157, 158, 164–165, *165*
bell peppers, 42, 43, 253, 267, 298. *See also* red peppers
orange peppers, 43
red peppers, 30, 88, *134*, 135, 138, 146–147, *147*, 151, 205, 253, 267
yellow peppers, 30, 43
berries, 190, 321, 323, 349
Antioxidants on the Run, *326*, 327, 346–347, *347*
Fruit Compote, 300, 301, 313, 314. *See also specific berries*
Bessinger, Jeannette, 14–17, 18–20, 48, 119, 139, 158, 198, 214, 216, 218, 333, 343
beta 1,3 glucan, 306
beta-carotene, 118, 215, 272
beta-cryptoxanthin, 253
betaine, 157
beta-sitosterol, 137
Better Than Bouillon, 297
beverages, 326–349. *See also* alcohol; *specific beverages*
Alkalizer, the, *326*, 327, 338, *338*
Antioxidants on the Run, *326*, 327, 346–347, *347*
Frozen Tropical Treat, *326*, 327, 342–343, *343*
functional, 345
green drinks, 332–333
green tea, 309
Hunger Buster, *326*, 327, 340, *340*
Jonny's Recipe for Supermarket SuperJuice, *326*, 327, 338
lemon water, 309
Liquid Polymeal Formula, *326*, 327, 339
Melon Snap, *326*, 327, 344, *344*
Nut Power, *326*, 327, 344, *344*
Sultry Summer Sangria, *326*, 327, 336–337, *337*
Sweet Morning Eye Opener, *326*, 327, *340*, 340
water, 328, 353
Bibb lettuce, 267
Black Bean Cakes, *24*, 25, 27, 34–35, *35*
black beans, *24*, 25, 27–29, 34–35, *35*, 43, 297, 300, 301, 307, 318–319, *319*, 322
black cherry juice, *326*, 327, 332, 338, 349
black pepper, 65, 151, 171, 191, 211, 249, 266, 296, 322
black peppercorns, 65, 249
black tea, 309, 341
black truffle oil, 274
blackberries, 309
blackstrap molasses, 171, 174, 176, 191, 211
blindness, 272
bloating, 76
blood oranges, 38
blood pressure, 50, 196, 270, 305, 306, 352–353
blood sugar, 13, 19, 27, 28, 30, 61, 70, 110, 111, 139, 157, 248, 252–253,

305–306, 329, 352–353. *See also* diabetes; glycemic index; insulin
blue green algae, 332, 333
blueberries, 41, 352
bok choy, 300, 301, 315. *See also* Chinese cabbage
bone health, 197, 218, 352–353
bouquet garni, 183, 249
Bowden, Jonny, 18, 19, 20, 21
brain health, 69, 70, 71, 158, 177, 215, 274
braising, 250–251
Brazil nuts, 352
breakfast dishes. *See also* smoothies
    Flax Pancakes, 300, 301, 303–304, 312–313, *313*
    Fruit Compote, 300, 301, 313, 314
breast cancer, 29, 95, 98, 157, 272, 273, 303, 306, 330
Brewer's yeast, 88
broccoli, 42, 156, 171, 217–218, 267, 273–274, 298, 309, 332, 352
    cardiovascular health and, 195
    Roasted Brussels Sprouts, Asparagus, and Broccoli with Toasted Hazelnuts, *212*, 213, 215, 217, 218, 230–231, *231*
    Steamed Green Veggies and Nuts, *244*, 245, 258–259, *259*
broccoli rabe, 45, 48, 50, 60–61, *61*, 65
Broccoli Rabe with Raspberry-Vinegar Reduction, *44*, 45, 48, 50, 60–61, *61*
Broiled Salmon with Tamari-Orange Marinade, *66*, 67, 69, 80–81, *81*
bromelain, 139
broth, 65, 89, 97, 113, 171, 191, 205, 211, 266, 297, 322
brown rice, *244*, 245, 251–253, 264–265, *265*, 266, *268*, 269, 290–291, *291*, 309, 353
Brussels sprouts, 156, *212*, 213, 215, 217–218, 230–231, *231*, 352
buckwheat, 309
Budoff, Matthew, 196
buffalo, *192*, 193, 195, 198, 202–203, *203*, 211, 253
Burr, George, 69
Burr, Marilyn, 69
butter, 12, 13, 89, 103, 113, 191, 211, 219, 266, 356–357. *See also* nut butters

C

C. botulinum, 274
cabbage, 42, 129, 155–157, 171, 249, 352. *See also* specific varieties of cabbage
cacao, 14, 50–51, 62–63, 65, 113, 197, 211. *See also* chocolate; cocoa
Caesar Salad, *268*, 269, 277, 294–295, *295*
calcium, 48, 138, 175, 176, 177, 197, 272, 305, 307
Calf's Liver and Green Onions, *152*,

153, 154–155, 158, 162–163, *163*
calories, portions and, 150
cancer, 13, 28–29, 47, 48, 71, 74, 117, 138, 196, 253, 271, 352–353. *See also specific types of cancer*
    alcohol and, 330
    aspartame and, 159
    beans and, 28–29, 306
    fats and, 49
    fermented foods and, 306
    fiber and, 111
    flaxseed oil and, 157
    fruit and, 98, 331, 332
    garlic and, 196, 251, 253, 271, 306
    grilling and, 47
    indoles and, 217, 249
    insulin and, 329
    isoflavones and, 306
    isothiocyanates and, 217
    lentils and, 306
    lignans, 303
    liver and, 155
    meat and, 46
    monounsaturated fats and, 137
    pectin and, 248
    phytochemicals and, 137, 217, 218, 341
    polyphenols and, 341
    pomegranates and, 174, 331
    quercetin and, 178, 195, 248
    resveratrol and, 271
    saponins and, 215
    sinigrin and, 218
    sulfur compounds and, 249
    turmeric and, 94, 95, 275
    vegetables and, 156, 194, 217, 251, 253, 273–274, 306
Candida albicans, 117
canola oil, 354–355
cantaloupe, 131, *326*, 327, 344, *344*, 352
capers, 151, 266
capric acid, 117, 276
capsaicin, 139, 253
caraway seeds, 249, 266
carbohydrates, 27, 29, 99, 159, 219, 329. *See also* sugars
carcinogens. *See* cancer
cardamom, 43, 133, 296, 322
cardiovascular health, 8, 13, 50, 70–71, 77, 117, 119–120, 136, 155–157, 196–197, 218, 275, 352–353
    ACE inhibitors and, 305
    alcohol and, 329
    apples and, 177, 195
    beans and, 251
    beets and, 157
    broccoli and, 195
    eggs and, 158
    fermented foods and, 248
    fiber and, 111
    flax and, 303
    garlic and, 196, 251, 270–271, 306
    insulin and, 329
    liver and, 155

natto and, 306
    onions and, 195, 251, 306
    pears and, 177
    pomegranates and, 174–175, 331
    quercetin and, 178
    red wine and, 177
    tea and, 195
carnitine, 345
carob, 309
carotenoids, 74, 118, 137, 215, 253, 272, 304
Carpender, Dana, 303
carrots, 129, 171, 267, 298, 323, *326*, 327, 338, *338*, *340*, 340, 349, 352
carvacrol, 253
cashews, 211, *268*, 269, 271, 272, 273, 276, 284–285, *285*, 298, 309, 348, 352
catfish, 121
cauliflower, *172*, 173, 176–177, 178, 184–185, *185*, 191, 274, 352
Cauliflower "Cream", *172*, 173, 176–177, 178, 184–185, *185*
cayenne pepper, 113, 133, 139, 151, 296
celery, 42, 171, 216, 298, 309, *326*, 327, 338, *338*, 349, 352
celery seed, 183
cereal, 190
cervical cancer, 98, 272
chard, 156, *192*, 193, 195, 197, *205*, 205–206, 211, 300, 301, 315, 353
charities, 239
cheese, 18, 65, 309. *See also specific cheeses*
chemoprotective action, 196
cherries, 42, 113, 174, 189, 191, 309, 332, 349, 352
cherry juice, 323, *326*, 327, 332, 338, 349
cherry tomatoes, 211
chervil, 183
chestnuts, 211, 309, 352
chicken, 88, 174, 191, 198, 285, 298, 309
    cage-free, 277
    free-range, 179, 277
    Persian-Style Chicken with Walnut, Onion, and Pomegranate Sauce, *172*, 173, 174, 178, 182–183, *183*
    Schlemmertopf-Roasted Pesto Chicken, *268*, 269, 270, 276, 280–281, *281*
    Slow-Cooker Chicken Curry, 273–274, 275, 288–289, *289*
chicory, 282–283, *283*, 298
chili, 133, *268*, 269, 271–273, 276, 284–285, *285*
chili peppers, 133, 253, 267, 352
chili powder, 296
Chinese cabbage, 88, 300, 301, 315
Chinese medicine, 94, 95, 197
chives, 183, 191, 249
chocolate, 51, 131, 197, 309. *See also* cacao; carob; cocoa
    dark, 9, 14, 51

Raw Chocolate Fondue, *90*, 91, 98, 108–109, *109*
Real-Food Brownies, 45, 50, 62–63, *63*
Silken Chocolate Parfaits, *192*, 193, 198, 208–209, *209*
cholesterol, 118, 352–353
    in eggs, 158
    fermented foods and, 306
    fiber and, 110, 111
    flavonoids and, 332
    garlic and, 196, 270–271
    HDL cholesterol, 70, 196
    LDL cholesterol, 158, 175, 196, 332
    metabolizing, 177
    monounsaturated fats and, 137
    National Cholesterol Education Program, 29
    pectin and, 248
    pomegranate and, 175
    in pumpkin seeds, 307
    saponins and, 215
choline, 158, 215, 304
Chopra, Deepak, 95
cilantro, 43, 95, 113, 133, 183, 296
cinnamon, 65, 113, 133, 190, 191, 194, 198, 211, 249, 296, 322, 348
circulation, 139, 196, 253, 329
Citrus Avocado Salad with Nut Oil, *24*, 25, 29, 38–39, *39*, 215
citrus fruits, 43
    Citrus Avocado Salad with Nut Oil, *24*, 25, 29
    Citrus-Stuffed Herbed Turkey, *212*, 213, 218, 224–225, *225*
    Sultry Summer Sangria, *326*, 327, 336–337, *337*
Citrus-Stuffed Herbed Turkey, *212*, 213, 218, 224–225, 228–229
CLA. *See* conjugated linolenic acid (CLA)
cloves, 87, 89, 191, 296
Coastal Alliance for Aquaculture Reform, 74
cocoa, 51, 62–63, 65, *90*, 91, 98, 108–109, *109*, 197, 211. *See also* cacao; chocolate
coconut extract, 209
coconut milk, *90*, 91, 95, 97, 106–107, *107*, 113, *114*, 115, 119, 130–131, *131*, 133, 298, 348
coconut oil, 12, 116–117, 118, 119, 133, 211, 348, 356–357
coconuts, *114*, 115, 116–117, 119, 126–127, *127*, 133, 275–276, 298, 348, 352. *See also* coconut extract; coconut milk; coconut oil
cod, 293
coffee, 42, 309
colds, alcohol and, 329
colorectal cancer, 46, 94, 117, 196, 249, 271, 272, 275
coloring agents, 74
condiments, 43. *See also* herbs; *specific condiments*; spices
Confetti Basmati Rice, *24*, 25, 30,

36–37, *37*
conjugated linolenic acid (CLA), 49
Conklin, Sarah, 71
constipation, fiber and, 110, 111
cookies, *152*, 153, 158, 168–169, *169*
cookware, 19, 35, 281, 343
Copp, Suzanne, 351
copper, 176, 251, 305
CoQ10, 345
coriander, 95, 138, 183, 249, 296
corn, 42, 309
coronary artery disease, 137
cottage cheese, 190, 309
cranberries, 216–217, 309, 331, 349, 352
   canned, 219
   cranberry juice, *326*, 327, 331, 338, 349
   Cranberry-Orange Relish, *212*, 213, 215, 216–217, 218, 234–235, *235*
   Holiday Waldorf Salad, *212*, 213, 215, 216, 218, 232–233, *233*
cranberry juice, *326*, 327, 331, 338, 349
Cranberry-Orange Relish, *212*, 213, 215, 216–217, 218, 234–235, *235*
cravings, 190
Creutzfeldt-Jakob Disease (vCJD), 155
crimini mushrooms, 251, 267
cruciferous vegetables, 274. *See also specific vegetables*
Crunchy Coconut Fruit Salad, *114*, 115, 116, 119, 126–127, *127*
cucumbers, *326*, 327, 338, *338*, 349
cumin, 43, 95, 113, 183, 249, 296
curcumin, 94
curcuminoids, 94, 274–275. *See also* curry; turmeric
Curried Quinoa Greens with Coconut Dressing, *90*, 91, 95, 97, 106–107, *107*
curry, 94, 95, 113, 125, 274–275. *See also* curcuminoids
   Curried Quinoa Greens with Coconut Dressing, *90*, 91, 95, 97, 106–107, *107*
   curry paste, *114*, 115, 118, 119, 124–125, *125*, 133
   curry powder, *90*, 91, 94–95, 97, 106–107, *107*, 113, 125, 183, 273–275, 288–289, *289*, 296
   Slow-Cooker Chicken Curry, 273, 274, 275, 288–289, *289*
   Thai-Spiced Mango and Prawns, *114*, 115, 118, 119, 124–125, *125*
curry paste, *114*, 115, 118, 119, 124–125, *125*, 133. *See also* curry
curry powder, *90*, 91, 94–95, 97, 106–107, *107*, 113, 125, 183, 273–275, 288–289, *289*, 296. *See also* curry

D

dairy products, *see specific dairy products*
D'Ambrosio, Steven, 137

dandelion greens, *66*, 67, 76–77, 84–85, *85*, 89, 352
Dandelion Greens with Warm Sesame Dressing, *66*, 67, 76, 77, 84–85, *85*
dates, 62–63, 65, 211, 309
Deepok Chopra Center, 196
defrosting, 112
Delicious Dal, *90*, 91, 102–103, *103*
desserts, 50, 214–216, 219
   Baked Apples, *172*, 173, 177, 178, 188–189, *189*
   cookies, *152*, 153, 158, 168–169, *169*
   fondue, *90*, 91, 98, 108–109, *109*
   Grilled Pineapple, *134*, 135, 139, 148–149, *149*
   Holiday Waldorf Salad, *212*, 213, 215, 216, 218, 232–233, *233*
   poached fruit, 72
   Raw Chocolate Fondue, *90*, 91, 98, 108–109, *109*
   Real-Food Brownies, 45, 50, 62–63, *63*
   Silken Chocolate Parfaits, *192*, 193, 198, 208–209, *209*
   sorbets, *66*, 67, 77, 86–87, *87*
   Spiced Pear Sorbet, *66*, 67, 77, 86–87, *87*
   Strawberry Soup, 30, 40–41
   Sweet and Simple Almond Butter Apricot Cookies, *152*, 153, 158, 168–169, *169*
   Sweet Potato Pie with Almond Oat Crust, *212*, 213, 214–215, 218, 236–238, *237*
   Tropical Frosties, *114*, 115, 119, 130–131, *131*
detoxification, 76, 95, 139, 176, 253, 272, 304
DHA (docosahexaenoic acid), 69, 70, 71, 73. *See also* omega-3 fatty acids
diabetes, 13, 71, 111, 137, 251, 329
diallyl sulfide, 195
Diet Plate, the, 150
diet soda, 159
Dietary Guidelines Advisory Committee, 71
diets. *See also* weight control
   Atkins diet, 13
   low-carb diets, 29
   low-fat diets, 12, 29, 99
   Mediterranean diet, 29, 136, 271, 306
   Western diet, 46
digestive system, 95, 111, 138, 196, 216, 248, 253, 273, 306, 352–353
Dijon mustard, 65, 89, 266, 296
dill, 138, 183, 296
diosgenin, 306
dips, *134*, 135, 138, 146–147, *147*. *See also* salsa
docosahexaenoic acid (DHA). *See* DHA (docosahexaenoic acid)
dopamine, 71
dressings, 85, 199. *See also* salads
Dutch ovens, 183

E

E. coli, 49
E3 Live, 333
eggplant, 293, 298
eggs, 13, 18, 65, 118, 158, 171, 179, 215, 277, 296, 304, 322, *326*, 327, 346–347, *347*, 348, 352
eicosapenaenoic acid (EPA). *See* EPA (eicosapenaenoic acid)
ellagic acid, 48, 332
endive, *192*, 193, 196, 197, 198, 206–207, *207*, 211
energy, 155, 210
energy bars, 11, 210
Enig, Mary, 354
Environmental Protection Agency (EPA), 121
Environmental Working Group, 42, 195
enzymes, 98, 138, 139, 176, 195, 272, 306
EPA (eicosapenaenoic acid), 70–71, 73. *See also* omega-3 fatty acids
Equal, 159
erectile dysfunction, 13, 50, 174–175
erythritol, 64
escarole, 282–283, *283*, 298
esophageal cancer, 194, 273
estrogen, 217
eugenol, 198
Extra Fiber, 348
eye health. *See* vision
eyes. *See* vision

F

factory farms, 47, 49, 99, 179, 247
fats, 14, 17, 19, 59, 99, 348. *See also* butter; fatty acids; ghee; low-fat diets; oils
   in avocados, 136–137
   in beef, 198
   cancer and, 49
   capric acid, 276
   in coconut, 116–117
   in eggs, 158, 215
   healthy, 69
   in lamb, 247, 257
   lauric acid, 276
   in meat, 219
   medium-chain triglycerides (MCTs), 117
   monounsaturated fats, 29, 136–137, 158, 218, 247, 253, 271
   in olive oil, 136–137
   in olives, 136–137
   reducing, 169
   in salmon, 69
   saturated fats, 117
   versus sugars, 13
   trans fats, 99, 271, 355
   in turkey, 218
   in venison, 250
fatty acids, 47, 49, 69–71, 73–75, 88, 120–121, 136, 167, 198, 303, also *specific fatty acids*
FDA. *See* Food and Drug Administration (FDA)

fennel, 183, 249, 296, 298
fermented foods, 248–249, 306, 307
feta cheese, 48
fiber, 14, 17, 19, 28, 48, 63, 76–77, 98, 110–111, 119, 156, 197, 210, 215, 218, 251, 307
Fiber One, 111
FiberSmart, 348
Fife, Bruce, 117
figs, 309, 352
filberts, 298
fines herbes, 183, 249
finishing oils, 274
fish, *see also specific fish*, 9, 17, 29, 136, 270, 352
   food safety and, 120–121, 132
   herbs for, 138
   mercury in, 120–121
   omega-3 fatty acids in, 120–121
   protein in, 120–121
   spices for, 138
   wild versus farm raised, 74–75, 99
fish oils, 354, 356–357
flavonoids, 10, 50, 119, 138, 177–178, 195, 248, 331–332
flavonols, 50, 51
flavorings, 113, 171, 194, 209, 211, 266, 322. *See also* condiments; herbs; seasonings; *specific extracts*; spices
Flax Pancakes, 300, 301, 303–304, 312–313, *313*
flaxseed, 69, 71, 88, 190, 300, 301, 303–304, 312–313, *313*, 322, 348, 352. *See also* flaxseed oil
flaxseed oil, 71, *152*, 153, 155, 156–157, 158, 166–167, *167*, 171, 348, 354, 356–357
flour, 19, 163, 171, 216, 250, 266, 309
folate. *See* folic acid (vitamin B9)
folic acid (vitamin B9), 155, 157, 177, 196, 197, 330
fondue, *90*, 91, 98, 108–109, *109*
Food and Drug Administration (FDA), 30, 42, 73, 132, 179
food preparation, 21, 47, 55, 56–57, 72, 99, 112, 215, 250–251, 332. *See also* food safety
food safety, 112, 120–121, 132, 224, 277. *See also* food preparation
Fragrant Chard, *192*, 193, 195, 197, *205*, 205–206
Franco, Oscar, 9, 14
free radicals, 155, 156, 272, 355
free-range labels, 179
fried foods, 99
Frozen Tropical Treat, *326*, 327, 342–343, *343*
Fruit Compote, *see also specific fruits*, 300, 301, 313, 314
fruits, 17, 18, 29, 109, 178, 349. *See also* juices
   Citrus Avocado Salad with Nut Oil, *24*, 25, 29
   citrus fruits, 38, 43, *212*, 213, 218, 224–225, *225*. *See also specific fruits*

dried fruits, 11, 174, 190. *See also specific fruits*
fiber in, 110
Frozen Tropical Treat, *326*, 327, 342–343, *343*
Fruit Compote, 300, 301, 313, 314
Liquid Polymeal Formula, *326*, 327, 339
preparation of, 72
Raw Chocolate Fondue, *90*, 91, 98, 108–109, *109*
Silken Chocolate Parfaits, *192*, 193, 198, 208–209, *209*
Sultry Summer Sangria, *326*, 327, 336–337, *337*
Tropical Frosties, *114*, 115, 119, 130–131, *131*
tropical fruits, 125. *See also specific fruits*
frying, 99
functional foods and beverages, 345

G
Gaby, Alan, 88
gallstones, alcohol and, 329
game meat, 253. *See also* meats
game meats, 99. *See also* venison
garbanzo beans, 65, 88
garlic, 9, 17, 35, 43, 65, 113, 133, 151, 194–196, 211, 218, 250–251, 253, 266, 270–273, 296, 306, 309, 322, 352. *See also* onions
  blood pressure and, 196
  Broccoli Rabe with Raspberry-Vinegar Reduction, 60–61
  cancer and, 196
  cardiovascular health and, 196
  cholesterol and, 196
  garlic powder, 266, 297
  garlic presses, 35
  garlic scapes, 60–61
  homocysteine and, 196
  preparation of, 105
  roasting, 139
  triglycerides and, 196
gastrointestinal cancer, 273
geraniol, 198
Ghandi, Mahatma, 303
ghee, 103, 113, 356–357
ginger, 87, 89, 113, 183, 194, 196, 211, 216, 249, 297, 322, 348
ginger brandy, 348
ginger juice, 89
gingerdiones, 196
gingerols, 196
gingko, 345
gingko tea, 345
Gironda, Vince, 332
Gittleman, Ann Louise, 118
glucose, 13. *See also* blood sugar
glutathione, 155, 304
glutathione-S-transferase, 195
gluten-free recipes, 158, 168–169
glycation, 250
glycemic index, 64, 159. *See also* blood sugar

goat cheese, 48
goji berries, 177, 178, 189, 191
gourmet salt, 113
grains, 37, 110, 291, 295. *See also* seeds; *specific grains*
Grand Marnier, 113
granola, 190
grape juice, 331–332
grapefruit, 149, 309, 352
grapes, 14, 42, *114*, 115, 116, 119, 126–127, *127*, 133, 156, 216, 309, 331–332, 352
grapeseed oil, 355
grasses, 332
great northern beans, 322
green beans, 89, 177, 191, 267, 298, 309
  Haricot Verts with Pomegranate Mint, *172*, 173, 177, 178, 186–187, *187*
  Steamed Green Veggies and Nuts, *244*, 245, 258–259, *259*
  Wild Rice and Green Beans with Shiitake Sauté, *66*, 67, 77, 82–83, *83*
green drinks, 332–333
green onions, *152*, 153, 154–155, 158, 162–163, *163*, 171, 191, 194, 211. *See also* scallions
green peppercorns, 183, 249
green tea, 197, 309, 341, 352
greens, 196, 265, 323. *See also* lettuce; salads; *specific greens*
  nutrients in, 138
  seasoning, 315
  Steamed Seasonal Greens, 300, 301, 315
  steaming, 315
  Sweet Beets and Greens, *152*, 153, 157, 158, 164–165, *165*
Grilled Pineapple, *134*, 135, 139, 148–149, *149*
grilling, 47, 55, 56–57
growth, 177
guava, 352

H
H. pylori, 249
Haas, Elson, 139
habenera, 297
hacho miso, 307
haddock, 293
halibut, *268*, 269, 271, 273, 276, 292–293, *293*, 299
hamburger. *See* beef
handwashing, 132
haricot verts, *172*, 173, 177, 178, 186–187, *187*, 191. *See also* green beans
Haricot Verts with Pomegranate Mint, *172*, 173, 177, 178, 186–187, *187*
Hato Mugi, 321
hay fever, quercetin and, 195
hazelnut extract, 209
hazelnut oil, 274
hazelnuts, 151, *212*, 213, 215, 217,

218, 230–231, *231*
HCA. *See* heterocyclic amines (HCAs)
HDL cholesterol, 70, 196
health bars, 11, 210
healthy cooking, 99
heart attack, 50. *See also* cardiovascular health
heart disease. *See* cardiovascular health
heartburn, turmeric and, 95
Heiss, Bob, 341
Heiss, Mary Lou, 341
hemoglobin, 112
hempseed oil, 356–357
hepatitis, 76, 95
herb teas, 309
herbs, 43, 65, 219. *See also* condiments; herb teas; *specific herbs*; spices
  for beef, 249
  bouquet garni, 183, 249
  Citrus-Stuffed Herbed Turkey, *212*, 213, 218, 224–225, *225*
  fines herbes, 183, 249
  for fish, 138
  for lamb, 249
  Lemon-Herb Salad, *268*, 269, 282–283, *283*
  for poultry, 183
  for red meat, 249
  vegetables and, 315
  for venison, 249
heterocyclic amines (HCAs), 56–57
Hibbeln, Joseph, 71
high-fructose corn syrup, 13, 219, 328, 331
holiday meals, 213–241
Holiday Waldorf Salad, *212*, 213, 215, 216, 218, 232–233, *233*
Homemade Energy Bars, 11
homocysteine, 155, 157, 196, 197, 304
honey, 30, 43, 64, 65, 89, 119, 133, 159, 174, 216, 219, 233, 267, 313
honeydew, *326*, 327, 344, *344*
hormones, 13, 19, 27, 28, 47, 49, 74, 99, 179, 217, 219, 247, 250, 303
horseradish, 249
hot peppers, 253, 267, 352
hot sauce, 151, 191, 297
humanely raised food, 18, 49, 163
Hunger Buster, *326*, 327, 340, 340

I
ice cream, 309
immune system, 117, 155, 178, 215, 218, 276, 305, 306
immunoglobins, 305
Indian medicine, 94, 196, 197. *See also* Ayurvedic medicine
indole-3-carbinol, 217
indoles, 156, 217, 249, 272
inflammation, 71, 248
Ingram, Cass, 253
insoluble fiber, 110
insulin, 13, 19, 27, 28, 157, 177, 307,

329, 331. *See also* blood sugar; diabetes
inulin, 76, 215
iodine, 175
Iowa Women's Health Study, 77, 177
iron, 47, 175, 176, 197, 250, 272
irritable bowel syndrome, fiber and, 111
isoflavones, 306
isothiocyanates, 217, 218, 273–274

J
jalapeño peppers, 267. *See also* chili peppers
jams, 65, 313
jicama, *114*, 115, 116, 118–119, 126–127, *127*, 129, 133
Job's Tears, 321
Jonny's Recipe for Supermarket SuperJuice, *326*, 327, 338
juices, 331–332. *See also specific juices*
  Jonny's Recipe for Supermarket SuperJuice, *326*, 327, 338
  Sweet Morning Eye Opener, *326*, 327, *340*, 340
juicing, 332
juniper berries, 249

K
Kalamata olives, *134*, 135, 139, 142–143, *143*, 151
kale, 107, 113, 272–273, 298, 332, 353
  asthma and, 88
  Curried Quinoa Greens with Coconut Dressing, *90*, 91, 95, 97, 106–107, *107*
  Turkey Chili with Cashews and Kale, *268*, 269, 271, 272, 273, 276, 284–285, *285*
kidney beans, 297
kimchee, 307. *See also* sauerkraut
king mackerel, 121
kiwifruit, 42, 98, 113, 133, 349, 353
  Crunchy Coconut Fruit Salad, *114*, 115, 116, 119, 126–127, *127*
  Sultry Summer Sangria, *326*, 327, 336–337, *337*
kohlrabi, 156
koji, 307
kudzu, 185, 191, 322

L
lactobacillus, 248
lamb, 247, 266, 309
  freezing, 257
  herbs for, 249
  Lamb Chops and Sauerkraut, *244*, 245, 247, 248–249, 256–257, *257*
  preparation of, 132, 257
  purchasing, 257
  spices for, 249
Lamb Chops and Sauerkraut, *244*, 245, 247, 248–249, 256–257, *257*
LaraBars, 210
lauric acid, 117, 276

Law, Malcolm, 8
LDL cholesterol, 158, 175, 196, 332
leeks, 194, 249, 267
legumes, 309. *See also* beans; lentils
lemon juice, 191, 267, 299
lemon pepper, 167, 171
lemon water, 309
lemon zest, 211, 267, 299
lemongrass, 138
Lemon-Herb Salad, *268*, 269, 282–283, *283*
lemons, 43, 151, 171, 263, 267, 309, 323, 349, 353
    lemon juice, 191, 267, 299
    lemon zest, 299
    Lemon-Herb Salad, *268*, 269, 282–283, *283*
    Sultry Summer Sangria, *326*, 327, 336–337, *337*
lentils, 29, *90*, 91, 102–103, *103*, 113, 306. *See also* beans; legumes
lettuce, 42, 43, 133, 191, 267, 309.
    See also arugula; chicory; endive; escarole; greens
    Bibb lettuce, *244*, 245, 262–263, *263*
    Caesar Salad, *268*, 269, 277, 294–295, *295*
    Romaine lettuce, 299
    Vinaigrette Salad, *244*, 245, 262–263, *263*
leukemia, 271
lignans, 303
lima beans, 309
lime juice, 113, 299
limes, 43, 113, 133, 299, 309, *326*, 327, 336–337, *337*, 349, 353
Liquid Polymeal Formula, *326*, 327, 339
liquid smoke, 266
listeria monocytogenes, 112
liver (organ meat), 154–155, 158, 171
    antioxidants in, 155
    Calf's Liver and Green Onions, *152*, 153, 154–155, 158, 162–163, *163*
    cancer and, 155
    cardiovascular health and, 155
    glutathione and, 304
liver health, 76, 95, 157, 272, *326*, 327, *338*, 338
Lo Han, 64, 159
low-carb diets, 29
low-fat cooking, 99
low-fat diets, 12, 29, 99
lung cancer, 178, 273
lutein, 77, 118, 137, 158, 197, 272, 304
lycopene, 253

M

maca powder, 348
Macadamia nut oil, 43, 65, 89, 171, 274, 323
mace, 183, 249
mackerel, 121
macular degeneration, 137, 272.
    See also vision

mad cow disease, 155
magnesium, 30, 48, 88, 119, 175, 176, 197, 305, 307
Majool dates, 63
mandolines, 129
manganese, 139, 175, 176, 177, 305, 307
mangoes, 42, 98, 113, 125, 133, 309, 349, 353
    Melon Snap, *326*, 327, 344, *344*, 344
    Thai-Spiced Mango and Prawns, *114*, 115, 118, 119, 124–125, *125*
marinades, *66*, 67, 69, 80–81, *81*, 199
marjoram, 138, 183, 249
"Master Cleanser," the, 139
Mayo Clinic, 110
mayonnaise, 219, 233
MCT oil, 339
MCTs. *See* medium-chain triglycerides (MCTs)
meats, 18, 42. *See also* poultry; *specific meats*
    Alzheimer's disease and, 46
    antibiotics in, 47, 49, 99
    braising, 250–251
    cancer and, 46
    chops, 132
    defense of, 46–47
    defrosting, 112
    E. coli and, 49
    factory farms and, 47, 49, 247
    fats in, 219
    food safety and, 112, 132
    game meat, 99, 253. *See also* venison
    grass-fed, 46, 47, 49, 99, 163, 198
    grilling, 47, 55, 56–57
    ground, 132
    herbs and, 249
    hormones in, 47, 49, 99
    humanely raised, 18, 49, 163
    iron in, 47
    marinating, 81
    organ meats, 155, 163
    organic, 46, 47, 49
    preparation of, 132, 163, *203*, 250–251, 253, 257
    roasts, 132
    spices and, 249
    steroids in, 47, 49, 99
Mediterranean diet, 29, 136, 271, 306
medium-chain triglyceride (MCT) oil, 339
medium-chain triglycerides (MCTs), 117, 275–276
melamine, 74
Melon Snap, *326*, 327, 344, *344*, 344
melons, 309, 349
    cantaloupe, 131, *326*, 327, 344, *344*, 344, 352
    honeydew, *326*, 327, 344, *344*
    Melon Snap, *326*, 327, 344, *344*
    watermelons, 131, 309, 353
mental health, 71
Mercola, Joe, 277
mercury, 120–121

metabolism, 155, 177
methemoglobin, 112
Mexican food, 41
milk, 42, 112, 309, 348
Miller, Sanford, 112, 132
millet, 309
minerals, 14, 17, 30, 77, 156, 218, 250, 272, 307. *See also specific minerals*
mini-meals, 170
mint, 43, 133, *172*, 173, 177, 178, 186–187, *187*, 191, 211, 249
miso, 300, 301, 306, 307, 318–319, *319*, 322
Miso Bean Soup, 300, 301, 307, 318–319, *319*
miso paste, 322
molasses. *See* blackstrap molasses
monocaprin, 117
monolaurin, 276
monounsaturated fats, 29, 136–137, 158, 218, 271
mood, 69, 71
morel mushrooms, 55
Morinda citrifolia fruit, 331
Mudd, Susan, 16, 351
mugi miso, 307
multivitamins, 355
mushrooms, 65, 267, 353
    crimini mushrooms, 251
    porcini mushrooms, 55
    Portobello Buffalo Tenderloin, *192*, 193, 195, 198, 202–203, *203*
    portobello mushrooms, *192*, 193, 195, 198, 202–203, *203*, 211
    shiitake mushrooms, *66*, 67, 77, 82–83, *83*, 89, 306, 323
    Wild Mushroom-Crusted Sirloin, 45, 46–47, 54–55, *55*
    Wild Rice and Green Beans with Shiitake Sauté, *66*, 67, 77, 82–83, *83*
mustard, 65, 183, 249, 296
    asian mustard, 89
    Dijon mustard, 65, 89, 266, 296
    mustard (dry), 171, 183, 191, 249
    mustard powder, 171, 249

N

natto, 306, 307
Navarre, Roy, 250
navy beans, 309
nectarines, 42
neural tube defects, 197
neurotoxins, aspartame and, 159
neurotransmitters, 197
niacin (vitamin B3), 247, 251
nitrates, 47
nitric oxide, 50
noni juice, *326*, 327, 331, 338, 349
nonstick cookware, 35
North Atlantic Treaty Organization (NATO), 71, 73
Nurses' Health Study, 29, 306
nut butters, *152*, 153, 158, 168–169, *169*, 171, *326*, 327, 344, 344, 348

nut milks, *326*, 327, 340, *340*, *344*, 344, 348. *See also* coconut milk
nut oils, 24, 25, 29, 43, 65, 89, 323. *See also specific nut oils*
Nut Power, *326*, 327, 344, *344*
nutmeg, 133, 183, 191, 322
Nutrasweet, 159
nutrition bars, 210
Nutrition Data, 155
nuts, 11, 29, 43, 48, 136, 189, 321, 323, 339, 348. *See also* coconuts; nut milks; nut oils; seeds; *specific nuts*
    fiber in, 110
    Steamed Green Veggies and Nuts, *244*, 245, 258–259, *259*
    toasting, 231

O

oats, 11, 110, 190, 191, *212*, 213, 214–215, 218, 236–238, *237*, 309, 322, 348, 353
obesity, 13, 71, 159, 329. *See also* weight control
oils, 55, 233, 274, 348, 354–355. *See also* fats; *specific oils*
oleic acid, 136
olive oil, 65, 89, 113, 136–137, 151, 171, 191, 211, 218–219, 253, 266, 270–271, 297, 306, 322, 353, 356–357
olives, *134*, 135, 136–137, 139, 142–143, *143*, 151, 267, 307
omega-3 fatty acids, 47, 49, 69, 70–71, 73–75, 88, 120–121, 157, 167, 198, 303, 355
omega-6 fatty acids, 167
omega-9 fatty acids, 136, 167
onion powder, 191
onions, 42, 43, 88, 113, 191, 194–196, 211, 250, 253, 267, 272–273, 299, 306, 309, 323, 353. *See also specific varieties of onions*
    allergies and, 88
    asthma and, 88
    cardiovascular health and, 195
    Persian-Style Chicken with Walnut, Onion, and Pomegranate Sauce, *172*, 173, 174, 178, 182–183, *183*
    pesticides and, 195
    preparation of, 105
    Steam-Baked Vidalia onions, *90*, 91, 97, 104–105, *105*
    sulfur compounds in, 195
oolong tea, 341
ORAC (oxygen radical absorbance capacity) test, 272
oral cancer, 137
orange extract, 113, 209
orange juice, 89, 323, 349
orange peppers, 43
oranges, 38, 43, 133, 216, 349, 353
    Cranberry-Orange Relish, *212*, 213, 215, 216–217, 218, 234–235, *235*
    Crunchy Coconut Fruit Salad, *114*, 115, 116, 119, 126–127, *127*

orange juice, 89, 323, 349
  Sultry Summer Sangria, *326*, 327, 336–337, *337*
oregano, 138, 249, 253, 266, *268*, 269, 282–283, *283*, 297
organ meats, 155, 163. *See also* liver (organ meat)
organic foods, 18, 42, 46, 47, 49, 132, 179, 219, 277, 337. *See also* antibiotics; artificial ingredients; hormones; pesticides; steroids
organicare labels, 179
osteocalcin, 138
osteoporosis, 156
oxidatation, 341
oxidation, 178
oxygen radical absorbance capacity (ORAC) test, 272

P
Page, Linda, 307
PAH. *See* polycyclic aromatic hydrocarbons (PAHs)
pain, capsaicin and, 253
PaleoGreens, 333
pancakes, 300, 301, 303–304, 312–313, *313*
pantothenic acid (vitamin B5), 251
pantry lists, 43, 65, 89, 113, 133, 151, 171, 191, 211, 266–267, 296–299, 322–323, 348–349
papayas, 42, 125, 309, 349, 353
paprika, 183, 191, 249
Parmesan cheese, 295, 296, 300, 301, 305, 316–317, *317*, 322
parsley, 43, 95, 151, 183, 266, 309, 348. *See also* cilantro
parsnips, 129
pasta, 309
pasteurization, 112
pastries, 309
PCBs, 74
peaches, 42, 190, 349, 353
peanut oil, 356–357
peanuts, 113, 298, 309, 353
pears, 42, 89, 190, 309
peas, 42, 267
pecans, 174, 191, 219, *244*, 245, 258–259, *259*, 267, 309, 348, 353
pectin, 248
Pedersen, Sue, 150
pepper. *See also* cayenne pepper; red pepper flakes
  black pepper, 65, 151, 171, 191, 211, 249, 266, 296, 322
  black peppercorns, 65, 249
  green peppercorns, 183, 249
  lemon pepper, 167, 171
  peppercorns, 65, 183, 249
  white pepper, 191
peppercorns, 65, 183, 249
peppers. *See* bell peppers; chili peppers
Perricone, Nicholas, 73
Persian-Style Chicken with Walnut, Onion, and Pomegranate Sauce, *172*, 173, 174, 178, 182–183, *183*

pesticides, 42, 74, 195, 219, 248
pesto, *268*, 269, 270, 276, 280–281, *281*
pH level, 308–309
phenols, 250–251
phenylalanine, 159
phosphatidylcholine, 158
phosphorus, 30, 250, 251, 276, 307
Physicians' Desk Reference, 117
phytic acid, 306
phytochemicals, 14, 17, 28, 137, 138, 156, 198, 215, 217–218, 249, 250–251, 272, 331. *See also* phytosterols; *specific phytochemicals*
phytosterols, 77, 137. *See also* phytochemicals
pickles, 307
pine nuts, 151, 323
pineapple juice, 349
pineapples, 42, 139, 151, 349, 353
  Grilled Pineapple, *134*, 135, 139, 148–149, *149*
  pineapple juice, 349
  preparation of, 149
  Sultry Summer Sangria, *326*, 327, 336–337, *337*
pinto beans, 309
Plain Brown Rice, *268*, 269, 290–291, *291*
plant foods, 99, 155. *See also* phytochemicals; phytosterols
PMS (premenstrual syndrome), 76
poaching, 72
pollock, 293
polycyclic aromatic hydrocarbons (PAHs), 56
polymeals, 8–11, 14, 17, 19, 20, *326*, 327, 330, 333, 339. *See also* smoothies; *specific recipes*
polyphenols, 10, 177–178, 197, 250, 329–330, 341
polypill, 8–9
polysaccharides, 306
pomegranate juice, 174, 191, 323, 331, 349
  Haricot Verts with Pomegranate Mint, *172*, 173, 177, 178, 186–187, *187*
  Persian-Style Chicken with Walnut, Onion, and Pomegranate Sauce, *172*, 173, 174, 178, 182–183, *183*
pomegranates, 174, 174–175, 175, 353. *See also* pomegranate juice
Pope, Tara Parker, 57
porcini mushrooms, 55
pork, 132, 309
port wine, 322
portions, calories and, 150
Portobello Buffalo Tenderloin, *192*, 193, 195, 198, 202–203, *203*
portobello mushrooms, *192*, 193, 195, 198, 202–203, *203*, 211
potassium, 30, 48, 77, 98, 119, 137, 139, 157, 175–177, 197, 215, 218, 250, 276, 305
potatoes, 19, 42, 177, 185, 219,

250–251, 267, 309. *See also* sweet potatoes
poultry, 42, 112, 132, 179, 183, 224, 270, 277, *285. See also* chicken; turkey
PowerBars, 210
prawns, *114*, 115, 118, 119, 124–125, *125*, 133. *See also* shrimp
pregnancy, 70, 120–121
premenstrual syndrome (PMS). *See* PMS (premenstrual syndrome)
proanthocyanidins, 331–332
probiotics, 30, 215, 248, 307. *See also* bacteria
produce, nutrients in, 250–251. *See also* fruits; herbs; *specific produce*; vegetables
prostate health, 29, 137, 157, 175, 248, 249, 303
protease inhibitors, 28, 306
protein, 10, 14, 17, 19, 30, 48, 120–121, 139, 155, 158, 210, 215, 218, 247, 250, 252, 270, 276, 307. *See also* protein bars; protein powder
protein bars, 210
protein combining, 265
protein powder, 304–305, 348
  Hunger Buster, *326*, 327, 340, *340*
  Liquid Polymeal Formula, *326*, 327, 339
  whey protein powder, 304–305, 323, *326*, 327, 342–343, *343*, *344*, 344, 348, 353
prunes, 309, 353
Pu-erh tea, 341
pumpkin, 219, 349, 353. *See also* squash
pumpkin seeds, 30, 43, 300, 301, 307, 320–321, *321*, 323, 339, 348

Q
Qi-Gong, 95
quercetin, 177–178, *178*, 195, 248
quinoa, 113, 252, 305, 309, 321, 322
  Curried Quinoa Greens with Coconut Dressing, *90*, 91, 95, 97, 106–107, *107*
  Quinoa Risotto with White Beans, Arugula, and Parmesan, 300, 301, 305, 316–317, *317*
Quinoa Risotto with White Beans, Arugula, and Parmesan, 300, 301, 305, 316–317, *317*

R
radishes, 129
raisins, 11, 299, 309
raspberries, 41, 50, 65, 211, 353
  Baby Spinach Salad with Fresh Raspberries, 45, 48, 58–59, *59*
  Broccoli Rabe with Raspberry-Vinegar Reduction, 45, 48, 50, 60–61, *61*
  raspberry jam, 65
raspberry jam, 65

Raw Chocolate Fondue, *90*, 91, 98, 108–109, *109*
raw foods, 99, 138, 145
Real-Food Brownies, *44*, 45, 50, 62–63, *63*
red beans, *244*, 245, 251–253, 264–265, *265*, 267
Red Beans, Brown Rice, and Lean Beef, *244*, 245, 251–253, 264–265, *265*
red lentils, 102–103, 113
red onions, 151, 267, 299, 323
red pepper flakes, 65, 297
red peppers, 30, 88, *134*, 135, 138, 146–147, *147*, 151, 205, 253, 267
red tea, 341
red wine, 9, 14, 17, 43, 65, 197, 211, 270–271, 297, 323, *326*, 327, 329–330, 336–337, *337*, 348
red wine vinegar, 267
reductions, 60–61
refried beans, 41
refrigeration, 132
relishes, *212*, 213, 215, 216–217, 218, 234–235, *235*
reproduction, 177
resveratrol, 14, 119, 271, 330
rhubarb, 309
riboflavin (vitamin B2), 155, 251
rice, 41, 43, 89, 252–253, 309, 322
  basmati rice, 25, 30, 36–37, 43, 296
  brown rice, *244*, 245, 251–253, 264–265, *265*, 266, *268*, 269, 290–291, *291*, 309, 353
  Confetti Basmati Rice, 30, 36–37, *37*
  glycemic impact of, 252–253
  Plain Brown Rice, *268*, 269, 290–291, *291*
  preparation of, 28, 83
  Red Beans, Brown Rice, and Lean Beef, *244*, 245, 251–253, 264–265, *265*
  rice milk, 190
  rice wine, 89
  Seeded Rice, 300, 301, 320–321, *321*
  storage of, 37
  varieties of, 252–253
  white, 19, 253
  wild rice, *66*, 67, 77, 82–83, *83*
  Wild Rice and Green Beans with Shiitake Sauté, *66*, 67, 77, 82–83, *83*
rice milk, 190
rice wine, 89
risotto. *See* quinoa; rice
Roasted Brussels Sprouts, Asparagus, and Broccoli with Toasted Hazelnuts, *212*, 213, 215, 217, 218, 230–231, *231*
Roasted Red Pepper Dip and Crudités, *134*, 135, 138, 146–147, *147*
Roasted Rutabaga Chips, *114*, 115, 119, 128–129, *129*, 139

Romaine lettuce, 299
rosemary, 183, 249
rosmarinic acid, 253
Rubman, Andrew, 104
Ruffner, Lora, 16, 177
rutabagas, *114*, 115, 119, 128–129, *129*, 133
rye, 309

S

saccharin, 159
safflower oil, 355
saffron, 183
sage, 138, 183, 249
sake, 89
salads, 205, 219
  Asparagus-Endive Salad, *192*, 193, 196, 197, 198, 206–207, *207*
  Baby Spinach Salad with Fresh Raspberries, 45, 48, 50, 58–59, *59*
  Broccoli Rabe with Raspberry-Vinegar Reduction, 60–61, *61*
  Caesar Salad, *268*, 269, 277, 294–295, *295*
  Citrus Avocado Salad with Nut Oil, *24*, 25, 29, 38–39
  Crunchy Coconut Fruit Salad, *114*, 115, 116, 119, 126–127, *127*
  Dandelion Greens with Warm Sesame Dressing, *66*, 67, 76, 77, 84–85, *85*
  Holiday Waldorf Salad, *212*, 213, 215, 216, 218, 232–233, *233*
  Lemon-Herb Salad, *268*, 269, 282–283, *283*
  Veggie Slaw with Flax Oil, *152*, 153, 156–157, 158, 166–167, *167*
  Vinaigrette Salad, *244*, 245, 262–263, *263*
salmon, 68–69, 71, 73, 118, 121
  asthma and, 88
  Broiled Salmon with Tamari-Orange Marinade, *66*, 67, 69, 80–81, *81*
  preparation of, 69
  wild versus farm raised, 74–75
salmonella, 277
salsa, 41, 43
salt, 43, 65, 113, 133, 151, 171, 175, 191, 211, 266, 297, 322
sangria, *326*, 327, 336–337, *337*
saponins, 28, 107, 215, 306
sardines, 88
saturated fats, 99, 117
sauerkraut, *244*, 245, 247, 248–249, 256–257, *257*, 267, 307
savory, 183, 249
scallions, 65, 89. *See also* green onions
Schlemmertopf pot, 19, 281
Schlemmertopf-Roasted Pesto Chicken, *268*, 269, 270, 276, 280–281, *281*
Schneider, Sally, 55
sea salt, 65, 89, 175

seafood, 81, 120–121. *See also* fish; shellfish; *specific types of seafood*
Sears, Barry, 27
seasonings, 89, 183, 297. *See also* condiments; flavorings; herbs; pepper; salt; spices
seed butters, 113. *See also* nut butters
seed oils, 133. *See also* nut oils
Seeded Rice, 300, 301, 320–321, *321*
seeds, 43, 231, 300, 301, 320–321, *321*, 339. *See also* almonds; grains; nuts; *specific seeds*
selenium, 120, 251, 276, 307
seltzer, 348
serotonin, 71, 197
sesame oil, 274, 356–357
sesame seeds, *66*, 67, 76, 77, 84–85, *85*, 89
sexually transmitted diseases, 117
shallots, 89, 165, 171
shellfish, 120–121, 309. *See also* specific types of shellfish
shiitake mushrooms, *66*, 67, 77, 82–83, *83*, 89, 306, 323
shogaols, 196
shrimp, 118, 125, 133. *See also* prawns
Silken Chocolate Parfaits, *192*, 193, 198, 208–209, *209*
sinigrin, 218
slaw, *152*, 153, 156–157, 158, 166–167, *167*
Slow-Cooker Chicken Curry, *268*, 269, 273, 274, 275, 288–289, *289*
smoothies, 190, 333, 337
  Alkalizer, the, *326*, 327, *338*, 338
  Antioxidants on the Run, *326*, 327, 346–347, *347*
  Frozen Tropical Treat, *326*, 327, 342–343, *343*
  Hunger Buster, *326*, 327, 340, *340*
  Jonny's Recipe for Supermarket SuperJuice, *326*, 327, 338
  Liquid Polymeal Formula, *326*, 327, 339
  Melon Snap, *326*, 327, 344, *344*
  Nut Power, *326*, 327, 344, *344*
  Sultry Summer Sangria, *326*, 327, 336–337, *337*
  Sweet Morning Eye Opener, *326*, 327, 340, *340*, 340
  tofu in, 199
snacks, 170, 190
sodium chloride, 175. *See also* salt
soft drinks, 159, 309
soluble fiber, 110
sorbets, *66*, 67, 77, 86–87, *87*
soups. *See also* stews
  broth, 65, 89, 113, 171, 191, 211, 266, 297, 322
  chili, *268*, 269, 271, 272, 273, 276, 284–285, *285*
  Miso Bean Soup, 300, 301, 307, 318–319, *319*
  raw, 145
  Spinach Soup, *134*, 135, 138, 139, 144–145, *145*

Strawberry Soup, 30, 40–41
Tangy Tomato Fish Stew, *268*, 269, 271, 273, 276, 292–293, *293*
Turkey Chili with Cashews and Kale, *268*, 269, 271, 272, 273, 276, 284–285, *285*
soy foods, 81, 83, 190, *192*, 193, 198–199, 208–209, *209*, 211, 300–301, 306–307, 318–319, *319*, 322, 348. *See also specific soy foods*
soy milk, 190, 306
soy sauce, 306
Spaghetti Squash, *268*, 269, 286–287, *287*, 306
Spanish olives, 267
spelt, 309
spice rubs, 50, 54, 55
Spiced Pear Sorbet, *66*, 67, 77, 86–87, *87*
spices, 43, 55, 65, 92–93, 196, 322. *See also* condiments; herbs; *specific spices*
  for beef, 249
  for fish, 138
  for lamb, 249
  medicinal properties of, 194
  for poultry, 183
  for red meat, 249
  spice rubs, 50, 54, 55
  Spiced Pear Sorbet, *66*, 67, 77, 86–87, *87*
  storage of, 55
  Thai-Spiced Mango and Prawns, *114*, 115, 118, 119, 124–125, *125*
  vegetables, 315
  for venison, 249
spinach, 42, 48, 65, 138, 151, 309, 332, 353
  asthma and, 88
  Baby Spinach Salad with Fresh Raspberries, 45, 48, 58–59, *59*
  food safety and, 132
  Spinach Soup, *134*, 135, 138, 139, 144–145, *145*
  Steamed Seasonal Greens, 300, 301, 315
  washing, 59
Spinach Soup, *134*, 135, 138, 139, 144–145, *145*
spirolina, 252
Splenda, 159
sprouted wheat bread, 309
squash, *268*, 269, 286–287, *287*, 299, 309. *See also* pumpkin
staphylococcus, 117
steak, 45, 46–47, 50, 54–55, *55*, 65
Steam-Baked Vidalia onions, *90*, 91, 97, 104–105, *105*
Steamed Green Veggies and Nuts, *244*, 245, 258–259, *259*
Steamed Seasonal Greens, 300, 301, 315
steel soap, 35
steroids, in meat, 47, 49, 99, 247
stevia, 64, 159, 323, 348
stews. *See also* soups

chili, *268*, 269, 271, 272, 273, 276, 284–285, *285*
Delicious Dal, *90*, 91, 102–103, *103*
Tangy Tomato Fish Stew, *268*, 269, 271, 273, 276, 292–293, *293*
Turkey Chili with Cashews and Kale, *268*, 269, 271, 272, 273, 276, 284–285, *285*
Venison Stew, *244*, 245, 250–251, 260–261, *261*
Stoll, Andrew, 71, 73
stomach cancer, 196, 271
strawberries, 30, 40–43, 98, 113, 211, *326*, 327, 346–347, *347*, 349, 353
Strawberry Soup, *24*, 25, 30, 40–41, *41*
Striped Bass with Sun-Dried Tomato and Kalamata Paste, *134*, 135, 139, 142–143, *143*
stroke, 50, 120, 157, 196, 329. *See also* cardiovascular health
stuffing, 219
substance P, 253
sucanat, 19
sucralose, 159
sugar alcohols, 64
sugarcane, 176
sugars, 13, 19, 63, 65, 99, 125, 176–177, 210, 219, 307, 328–329, 331. *See also* blackstrap molasses; blood sugar; sweeteners
sulfides, 195, 249
sulforaphane, 176, 218, 272, 274
sulfoxides, 195, 249
sulfur compounds, 195, 249
Sultry Summer Sangria, *326*, 327, 336–337, *337*
sun-dried tomatoes, *134*, 135, 139, 142–143, *143*, 151, 299
sunflower seeds, 300, 301, 320–321, *321*, 348, 353
Super Liquid Folate, 330
Sweet and Simple Almond Butter Apricot Cookies, *152*, 153, 158, 168–169, *169*
Sweet Beets and Greens, *152*, 153, 157, 158, 164–165, *165*
Sweet Morning Eye Opener, *326*, 327, 340, 340
Sweet 'n Low, 159
sweet onions, 299
Sweet Potato Pie with Almond Oat Crust, *212*, 213, 214–215, 218, 236–238, *237*
sweet potatoes, 129, *212*, 213, 214–215, 218, 219, *237*, 299, 309, 349, 353
sweeteners, 159, 171, 174, 215. *See also specific sweeteners*; sugars
sweets, 190. *See also* desserts
Swiss chard. *See* chard
swordfish, 121

T

tamari sauce, *66*, 67, 69, 80–81, *81*, 89
Tangy Tomato Fish Stew, *268*, 269, 271, 273, 276, 292–293, *293*
taraxacum officinale, 76
tarragon, 183, 249
Taubes, Gary, 13, 275
tea, 195, 197, 309, 341, 345, 352. *See also specific teas*
tempeh, 306
Thai red curry paste, 133
Thai-Spiced Mango and Prawns, *114*, 115, 118, 119, 124–125, *125*
Theobroma cacao, 51
thiosulfinates, 195, 249
thyme, 183, 249, 266
thymol, 253
tilefish, 121
tofu, 81, 83, *192*, 193, 198, 199, 208–209, *209*, 211, 306, 348
tomato paste, 267, 299
tomato sauce, 191
tomatoes, 113, 211, 253, 267, 299, 353
    cherry tomatoes, 211
    seeding, 103
    Striped Bass with Sun-Dried Tomato and Kalamata Paste, *134*, 135, 139, 142–143, *143*
    sun-dried tomatoes, *134*, 135, 139, 142–143, *143*, 151, 299
    Tangy Tomato Fish Stew, *268*, 269, 271, 273, 276, 292–293, *293*
    tomato paste, 267
toxins, fiber and, 111
trans fats, 99, 210, 271, 355
triglycerides, 70, 117, 118, 137, 196, 270–271, 275–276, 331
Tropical Frosties, *114*, 115, 119, 130–131, *131*
tropical fruit, 125
truffle oils, 274
tryptophan, 197, 216
Tschirky, Oscar, 216
tumors. *See* cancer
tuna, 121
turkey, 198, 216, 218, 266, 298, 309
    carving, 229
    choosing a, 218
    Citrus-Stuffed Herbed Turkey, *212*, 213, 218, 224–225, *225*, 228–229
    preparation of, 224–225, 228–229
    Turkey Chili with Cashews and Kale, *268*, 269, 271, 272, 273, 276, 284–285, *285*
turkey bacon, 211
Turkey Chili with Cashews and Kale, *268*, 269, 271, 272, 273, 276, 284–285, *285*
turmeric, 94–95, 113, 183, 274–275, 297. *See also* curcuminoids

Turner, Lisa, 88
turnips, 129
type 2 diabetes. *See* diabetes

U

ulcers, 249
Ulsheimer, Charles J., 250
ume plum vinegar, 297, 323
Underdonk, Christy, 11
urinary tract infections, 331
U.S. Department of Agriculture, 70
uterine cancer, 157, 303

V

vanilla almond milk, 113, *114*, 115, 119, 130–131, *131*, 133. *See also* almond milk
vanilla extract, 89, 113, 171, 211, 322
veal, preparation of, 132
vegetable juices, 309, *326*, 327, 340, *340*
vegetable oil, 65, 99
vegetables, 9, 17, 18, 29, 46, 136, 151, 178, *187*, 319, 349. *See also* beans; herbs; salads; *specific vegetables*
    Alkalizer, the, *326*, 327, 338, *338*
    Allium family, 194–196, 270–271. *See also* garlic; onions
    Brassica family, 156, 176–177, 217–218. *See also specific vegetables*
    cruciferous vegetables, 274. *See also specific vegetables*
    fiber in, 110
    food safety and, 132
    grilling and, 57
    pH level and, 308–309
    preparation of, 129
    raw vegetables, 138
    Roasted Red Pepper Dip and Crudités, *134*, 135, 138, 146–147, *147*
    seasoning, 315
    Steamed Green Veggies and Nuts, *244*, 245, 258–259, *259*
    Steamed Seasonal Greens, 315
    steaming, 258–259
    vegetable juices, 309, *326*, 327, *340*, 340
vegetarianism, 300
Veggie Slaw with Flax Oil, *152*, 153, 156–157, 158, 166–167, *167*
venison, *244*, 245, 249, 249–251, 260–261, *261*, 266
Venison Stew, *244*, 245, 250–251, 260–261, *261*
Vidalia onions, *90*, 91, 97, 104–105, *105*, 113, 194, 273
Vinaigrette Salad, *244*, 245, 262–263, *263*
vinegars, 156, 157, 274. *See also specific vinegars*
vision, 70, 77, 137, 158, 272, 304, 352–353
Vital Choice Seafood, 75

vitamin A, 30, 98, 155, 177, 197, 215, 253, 272
vitamin B12, 155, 196, 247, 330
vitamin B2 (riboflavin). *See* riboflavin (vitamin B2)
vitamin B3 (niacin). *See* niacin (vitamin B3)
vitamin B5 (pantothenic acid). *See* pantothenic acid (vitamin B5)
vitamin B6, 88, 155, 196
vitamin B9 (folic acid). *See* folic acid (vitamin B9)
vitamin C, 30, 48, 88, 253, 272. *See also* ascorbic acid
vitamin E, 118
vitamin K, 48, 138, 197, 218, 253, 272
vitamins, 14, 17, 156, 177, 250, 272, 306, 355. *See also* B vitamins; *specific vitamins*
Vita-Mix, 343
Volek, Jeff, 61, 157

W

Wald, Nicholas, 8
walnut oil, 356–357
walnuts, 174, 191, 216, 267, 309, 353
    Holiday Waldorf Salad, *212*, 213, 215, 216, 218, 232–233, *233*
    Persian-Style Chicken with Walnut, Onion, and Pomegranate Sauce, *172*, 173, 174, 178, 182–183, *183*
    Steamed Green Veggies and Nuts, *244*, 245, 258–259, *259*
Walters, Heather MacLean, 250
water, 328, 353
water chestnuts, 211, 299
water retention, 76
watercress, 211, *244*, 245, 262–263, *263*, 267, 353
watermelons, 131, 309, 353
weight control, 28, 111, 156, 214
wheat, 190, 309, 332, 333, 353
wheat bran, 353
wheat germ, 190, 353
wheatgrass, 332, 333
whey protein powder, 304–305, 323, *326*, 327, 342–343, *343*, 344, *344*, 344, *344*, 348, 353
white beans, 300, 301, 305, 316–317, *317*
"white" foods, 19
white pepper, 191
white rice, 253, 309
white tea, 341
white truffle oil, 274
white wine, 89, 267
white wine vinegar, 211
whole foods, 99
Wild Mushroom-Crusted Sirloin, *44*, 45, 46–47, 50, 54–55, *55*
wild mushrooms, *44*, 45, 46–47, 54–55, 65
wild rice, *55*, *66*, 67, 77, 82–83, *83*, 89, 309

Wild Rice and Green Beans with Shiitake Sauté, *66*, 67, 77, 82–83, *83*
Willett, Walter, 12
Wilshire, Regina, 16, 250, 251
wine. *See* Mediterranean diet; sangria; *specific varieties of wine*
Worcestershire sauce, 266, 297
wound healing, 177

X

xylitol, 64, 159, 169, 171, 190, 348

Y

yams, *326*, 327, *340*, 340, 349
yeast, 117
yellow onions, 299, 323
yellow peppers, 30, 43
yerba matte, 341
yogurt, 30, 43, 145, 190, 216, 219, 233, 296, 307, 309, 313, 322, 353

Z

zeaxanthin, 77, 137, 158, 197, 272, 304
zinc, 175, 247, 250, 251, 305, 307
zingerone, 196
Zone, the, 27
zucchini, 299, 309